Foreword by Dr A Stewart

OPPOSITE
WORLD

Your Guide To Everything That Matters

KYLIE STEWART

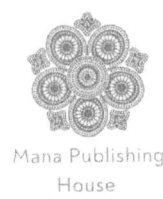

Mana Publishing House

First published by Mana Publishing House 2025

Copyright © 2025 Kylie Stewart

First edition

Edited by Dr Christina Marigold Houen of Perfect Words Editing

This book is written in Australian English.

Disclaimer: The information presented in this book is for educational and informational purposes only. It is not intended to substitute for professional medical, psychological or financial advice, diagnosis, or treatment. Always seek the advice of qualified professionals regarding any questions or concerns. The author and publisher disclaim any liability arising from using or misusing the information provided. This book references declassified information from publicly available sources. The author makes no claims beyond those documented in these sources and uses them solely for educational purposes.

DEDICATION

I want to dedicate this book to my beautiful loved ones, who have tolerated my head being in my computer for months. I also dedicate it to everyone who dares to step outside their programming and social norms to be the person their soul wants them to be.

FOREWORD

It's rare to find a book that challenges how we think and then inspires us to act. *Opposite World* does just that. It offers not just a collection of ideas but an invitation to see life through a new lens that empowers us to change our perspectives, confront our limitations, and reimagine what's possible. We have everything we need inside us, and this book will give you all the keys to unlock your powers.

The message behind *Opposite World* resonates so deeply with me. It's a book that doesn't just offer ideas; it reflects the essence of the life that Kylie has built for herself. A life rooted in conscious growth, intentional living, and constant transformation. I've had the unique privilege of witnessing this journey up close as her husband and someone who shares her deep commitment to personal development and well-being. The principles that Kylie writes about are not abstract theories to her; they are the guiding forces that have shaped her life, and through her words, they can also shape yours. The insights shared in *Opposite World* come from years of introspection, learning, and personal evolution. What's most striking to me is how Kylie not only talks about transformation, but lives it every day. Her life is a testament to the power of shifting perspective, of looking at life's challenges not as roadblocks but as opportunities for growth. She is someone who practises what she preaches. Her lifestyle approach to living with clarity, purpose, and vitality is a real-world example of the principles she beautifully captures in this book.

For over 30 years, I've had the privilege of working as an acupuncturist and doctor of Chinese medicine. Every day, I help people transform their physical and emotional well-being, often witnessing results that can only be described as miraculous. My work is grounded in a deep understanding of the body's interconnectedness, energy flow, and balance of systems. After doing over 150,000 treatments, I've come to realise that the true path to healing is never about merely fixing symptoms. It's about shifting how we see ourselves and the world around us, which takes us to the root cause. I see people recalibrate their perspectives to allow for a deeper understanding of their potential. There is a big difference between simply managing illness and pain and finding true restoration. We have the ability to access more power than we are led to believe — and for those who often wonder, is there more? Yes, there is.

This power includes learning, growing, and changing, regardless of age or past. You may have heard myths about the brain, like the idea that we can't grow new neurons or that all our information is stored in the brain alone. Science now proves otherwise. In fact, we can grow new neurons until the day we die (Eriksson et al., 1998)—it's a case of 'use it or lose it.' You'll discover more about this in the book as you explore how to unlock untapped potential so that true healing can take hold. What you will learn is that although your brain is powerful, your consciousness, the real you, is limitless.

This book is designed to change your perspective on many topics. It offers pathways that go beyond superficial changes, reaching deep into the transformation of your inner life. You can use this as a guide to break through your limitations, expand your awareness, and create a life of greater meaning and fulfilment.

What makes *Opposite World* special is that it offers not only insights but also actionable steps. This is not a book of theory; it's a book of lived wisdom. As someone who has been on this journey and working closely with people every day, I can say that true, lasting transformation doesn't come from a single moment of insight; it comes from a sustained effort to change how we approach life. It's about creating habits, mindsets, awareness, and practices that support our growth and well-being. I can tell you: the potential transformation presented in this book is not only possible, it's happening for people daily, in small, intentional steps.

As I've watched Kylie grow personally and professionally, I've been continually inspired by her ability to live a life of purpose and intention. I admire her unwavering commitment to personal evolution and her capacity to share that wisdom and deep understanding with others, whether talking with a friend or family member or coaching an individual on their own journey. Now, she is reaching out further by writing this book. I am incredibly proud of Kylie's work. I've seen how she's poured her heart and soul into these pages, and I believe wholeheartedly that *Opposite World* has the potential to change lives.

Whether you're just beginning your personal development journey or have been on this path for years, this book offers valuable insights to help you move to the next level. I encourage you to approach this book with an open mind and a willingness to embrace the possibility of change. It's a book that will challenge, inspire, and ultimately empower you to step into the life you've always wanted.

I am honoured to be a part of this book's journey and excited for you to embark on your own. Thank you for taking this step toward change. I know it will be a journey worth taking. Come join us in *Opposite World*.

— Dr. Andrew Stewart

TABLE OF CONTENTS

FOREWORD V

INTRODUCTION XIII

CHAPTER 1 - THE FIELD 19
    Exploring the Invisible Force Around Us 19
    A Universal Connection 21
    Breaking Down the Dense Science 25
    The Field Is Like a Boomerang 30
    Planetary Connections 31
    Have You Felt It? 32
    How Can I Tap into the Field? 35
    Could Children Learn to Tap into the Field? 35

CHAPTER 2 - A RESILIENT HEART 39
    Heart Coherence 39
    The Heart Is the Real Boss 41
    Coherence as a Collective 43
    What Science Says 44
    Live Through Your Heart 46

CHAPTER 3 - WHO AM I? 49
    The Mirror Within 49
    Self-Reflection 53
    The Many Aspects of You 56
    Know Thyself 60
    My Highest Values 64
    The Life Alignment Tracker 67
    Spotting the Bumpy Areas 68
    Money Mindset 70
    Romantic Relationships 72

CHAPTER 4 - UNMASKING THE SILENT SHADOWS WITHIN 77

    Letting the Light In 77
    What Are Emotions? 80
    The Connection Between Emotions and Health 82
    Distractions from Emotions 89
    Releasing Emotions – Feel it to Heal it 92
    R.E.L.E.A.S.E – A Tool for Letting Go 94
    To Cry or Not to Cry 96

CHAPTER 5 - THOUGHT SCULPTING 103

    It's Time to Change That Programming 103
    Thought–Emotion Loop 109
    Stepping into Neutrality: A Booster Step 110
    Chipping Away 112
    The Daily Thought-Sculpting Game 112
    The Principles of Polarity – Think to the Opposite 115

CHAPTER 6 - BE YOUR ALCHEMIST FOR TRANSFORMATION 121

    What is Alchemy? 121
    Changing Patterns 123
    Power of Forgiveness 124
    Alchemy: Transmuting Fear into Love 126
    Flow State 131
    Final Words on Alchemy 136
    Final Words on the Four Steps 136

CHAPTER 7 - THE LAYERS OF YOU 139

    Your Body and Mind 139
    Your Higher Self 141
    The Field 141
    Other Layers? 143
    Levels of Awareness 143
    Is This Your Only Life? 147

CHAPTER 8 - LIFE BY DESIGN 151
- Creating Your Dream Life 151
- The Science Backing Manifestation 154
- Creating Abundance 155
- Key Steps of Manifestation.. 156
- DREAM Your Reality.. 158
- When Is the Best Time to Create Your Dream Life?.................. 158
- Mars, Venus and Intention Setting... 159
- Avoiding the Pitfalls of Manifestation 159
- Plot Twist.. 162

CHAPTER 9 - MEDITATION 163
- The Benefits of Meditation 164
- What Science Says About Meditation 166
- How to Meditate... 168
- Energy Alignment Methods... 169
- Sound Frequencies... 172
- Heart and Brain Coherence... 174
- Matching the Frequency of Your Manifestations.................... 174
- Meditation Tips... 175
- The Power of Group Meditations 179
- Quiet Fields - The Power of Global Sleep Times 180
- Real-Life Stories from Regular Meditators 182

CHAPTER 10 - BIOHACKS FOR THE BODY 197
- Simple 'Free' Daily Biohacks 199
- My Biohacking Rituals 203

CHAPTER 11 - REALIGNING RELATIONSHIPS AS YOU TRANSFORM 207

Embracing Change While Others Stay the Same...................207
Protect Your Energy...................211
Stay on Your Bridge...................211
The Power of Saying No...................213
Moving Beyond Generational Limits...................214

CHAPTER 12 - YOUR ACTION BLUEPRINT 217

Your Tangible Plan...................220
Your Life Keys...................222
Resilience Insurance...................223

FINAL WORDS 227
ABOUT THE AUTHOR 229
RECOMMENDATIONS 231
REFERENCES 233

INTRODUCTION

Imagine living in a world where you possess superhuman abilities in body, mind, and spirit. A world so nourishing that you heal a little more every single day. Imagine a place where love and compassion ground your emotions rather than stress, anxiety, or loneliness, no matter what happens around you. A limitless world where you can design your dream life and tap into your intuition whenever you need to. Sounds like a sci-fi movie, right? Guess what? There is a place in this world for everyone, regardless of background, and it's not hidden in a galaxy far, far away; it's within you and is your birthright. The only requirement? You need to want it. This world awaits, and this book will guide you on your personalised bridge to get there.

You might think, 'I hope this isn't another self-help book promising rainbows and unicorns'. I am happy to tell you that this book isn't about surface-level platitudes or tips you'll forget by next Tuesday. Why will this be different? Because it takes a holistic approach that will cover all bases on your path to being your best self. It acknowledges that everyone starts from a unique place and may require a different path to reach their goals. You will receive simple guidance tailored to suit you rather than forcing a one-size-fits-all approach.

This book's simple structure gives you the knowledge you need and, more importantly, the tools to turn that knowledge into wisdom. After all, knowing something is one thing, but applying it is when the real transformation begins. People today are full of knowledge but starved of wisdom. How often have you witnessed people who seem to know a lot about human behaviour and self-awareness, yet don't embody what they preach? This widespread issue calls for an end to endless data collection; it's time to uncover true wisdom and embody it. I aim to combine the best teaching methods and simplify the dense wording. Reading many unfamiliar words is unproductive. It is my wish that you depart with both knowledge and wisdom.

After discovering this wisdom gap, I designed this book to help bring everything together. What do I mean by bridging everything together? Let's dive into this a little further. Many self-help books offer fantastic practical tips but often only speak to the left brain. So, people learn the lessons and try to take action, yet nothing changes how they feel. Why? Because those books don't speak to the true essence of who the readers are. Everyone is distinct and might need to address specific obstacles before engaging in these activities. On the flip side, many spiritual books offer profound insights into our universe but only speak to the right brain. The reader feels like they're *'spiritualling'* so hard (yes, that's not a proper word, but I like it), yet their life doesn't seem to change. Why? Because they're not getting the practical tools their left brain needs to run the show.

Have you heard the term spiritual bypassing? This term describes people who try to get above their negative emotions or traumas because they are too painful; they use spiritual modalities rather than meeting their suffering and working on it. It may work for a while, but they fall apart when they experience a significant setback or stop spiritualling. I like to think there is a lovely balance between the two styles, and I will guide you along this middle path. Let's be honest: most books in this space also lack humour and lightness, which I understand because some topics can be heavy. I want to bring this lightness because, let's face it, we have to laugh at ourselves sometimes. Also, I struggle to be serious for too long, so I'm probably amusing myself, if nothing else.

Here's how this book was conceived. I have wanted to write a book since I was very young, but I never knew quite what to write about; all I knew was that I wanted to help people. No, I don't think I'm Mother Theresa. Far from it! It's just one of my core values; we'll help you find yours, too. I did commence writing a book many years ago and ended up deleting it because I didn't wish for trauma to be my story. I now only feel a genuine love towards that story. People find this a little strange and expect I should have bitterness, but forgiveness is powerful, and we will delve into the science of that in Chapter 6. We all have stories, some more painful than others, but it's time to ditch them, as healing is possible for everyone. If you are ready to let go of a story or a way of thinking, you have come to the right place. Since I deleted that book, I have been putting the question out there for years on what I should write a book about. When I finally surrendered to this, left it in my higher self's hands, and stopped trying to find answers with my left brain, it all came to me in one gush. I was meditating at the time, so I pulled out the laptop amid 'Zen-like bliss' and typed for hours. I could not have written this book without many factors: the many random courses and degrees I have taken, the amazing people in my life, my fascination for human behaviour and some pretty dark experiences. I see the bigger picture; I now know the story — the story is that I no longer have a story. I share this because, as you journey through this book, I encourage you to let go of your story, surrender and trust that your best life awaits. Throughout this book, we will clear your path and connect you with your limitless potential.

You may be wondering why this book is titled *Opposite World*. The term *Opposite World* is one I have been saying either out loud or in my head for years. I have always felt this pull to do the opposite of what most people are doing. I thought I was just being rebellious, but I now know it's the key to unlocking everything. Don't worry; this will make sense as you work through this book. There will be times when you feel you are learning to walk backwards after a lifetime of marching forwards. Sometimes, we need to unlearn and see things from a new perspective.

We will discover some fascinating ancient truths, blending timeless wisdom with modern evidence-based science. After all, a little proof never hurts. You will also be given practical tools you can use in your life for self-exploration and self-transformation. It won't be complicated; it will be simple and practical. We will cover a lot, and you can choose the best path for you.

I designed this book's layout in a very deliberate order. Think of it as a well-planned feast for the soul, a life-changing buffet. I would encourage you to pause at each chapter (especially chapters 3 to 6) and spend the time to use the tools in your daily life. You can return to specific chapters as your life evolves; use this as your guide. Along the way, we will dive into exercises to truly get to know yourself, your values, your beliefs and even those sneaky hidden shadows you may realise you've been avoiding. Before we whip up lasting emotional change, we must shake up how we think and feel. It's all about learning the opposites and leaving your old self in the past. You may find some chapters familiar and some a little foreign. I want to meet you where you are at. Think of it as if you are coming to a new school, and you have already learnt some of the subjects in the curriculum and some you have not heard of, yet they are all essential to graduate. Once you understand all the subjects, you will have a solid foundation to become your stable truth. We have saved the best chapters to the end, and it's all about creating your best life. Consider this the dessert section of our buffet. It will be worth the wait.

In *Opposite World*, it's all about doing things differently. We will step outside our programming and open up to another way of being, doing and thinking. We will step outside our five senses; these senses are incredible yet limited. You will turn philosophy into your religion, and your understanding of reality will change forever. I want to give you a heads-up now. As you take this journey, your heart may open in ways you never thought possible. You might feel all soft and gooey inside, like a marshmallow over a campfire. But on the flip side, brace yourself — there may also be moments when you feel a little mad, like you want to toss the book across the room. Believe me, this is a good thing! Not the act of book throwing, but the emotions that may come up. Consider that your frustration may point to a hidden belief or inauthenticity. We may not need to analyse it; instead, we can embrace and dissolve it together.

Along with going through the four steps in this book, I will give you some profound keys. These keys reappear at the book's end; pick up the ones that resonate with you and let them guide you through your transformations. Make notes next to them if needed (for eBook or Audible users, all writing material can be downloaded from our website).

As you near the end of this book, you might notice your life and your perception of the world shifting. Everything and everyone around you feels so foreign. There is no need to panic! We're not about to tell you to pack your bags and become a monk (unless you want to). In Chapter 11, you'll receive advice you didn't even know you needed. Think of it as a survival guide for escaping the matrix, with strategies to help you adapt to the people around you. This chapter is my favourite, as I would have loved this advice, and I think there is a strong need for it.

I could have written an entire book on each chapter, but I wanted this book to be your simple guide. When you reach a section that resonates with you, I will point you toward true experts in the Field, whether other books or teachers. I hope to empower every reader to be the happiest and most powerful person they can be.

I honour you for reading this book instead of scrolling on your phone. The key to expansion is always to remain curious and always be in awe.

As Albert Einstein said, '*The important thing is to not stop questioning. Curiosity has its own reason for existing. One cannot help but be in awe when contemplating the mysteries of eternity, of life, and of the marvellous structure of reality. It is enough if one tries merely to comprehend a little of this mystery every day*'.

Let's explore *Opposite World*; you'll soon realise it's where the cool people hang out.

CHAPTER 1

THE FIELD

If you want to find the secrets of the universe, think in terms of energy, frequency and vibration. – Nikola Tesla

Exploring the Invisible Force Around Us

Have you ever met someone who seems different to most people, something you can't quite put your finger on, yet you're inexplicably drawn to them? They make you feel good just being around them. There's a particular mystery about them. An angelic energy infuses their powerful yet gentle nature. While they are seldom talkative, their words are profound. Their foresight, awareness and intuition seem mystic. Like all of us, they have had stressors and lead a busy life, but they always appear unaffected and calm. They are successful and abundant, yet humble. This person is in touch with their true self and lives authentically, free from societal programming. This person lives in *Opposite World* and is deeply in alignment with the Field. We will meet someone like this at the end of the book.

This chapter dives into the mystical energy surrounding us all, which, for simplicity's sake, we'll call the Field throughout the book. Have you ever sensed a silent knowing, a gentle push from deep within yourself, suggesting there is something more just beyond your reach? That's because there is — you just have to remember and unlearn some programming. What is the Field? I'll give you some visuals to help you understand it. Think of it as the Wi-Fi of the universe, an all-encompassing, invisible fabric that connects, permeates, and unites everything, including us; we are a thread within this fabric. Or imagine it as an invisible web stretching across the cosmos, connecting every star, every leaf and every heartbeat. It's not a place you travel to; it's an energy hidden from sight that has been there all along. Once you understand this force, you'll realise you have the power to change your life; it's a tool at your fingertips. The Field is always available, connecting you to infinite possibilities and empowering you to shape the life you desire. This book will combine ancient wisdom with modern science to explore the Field. While ancient traditions described it long ago, and quantum science is beginning to understand it, the Field remains beautifully mysterious.

Are you thinking this is crazy talk? Keep your mind open because we live in a world where we've been taught to rely only on what we can see, touch, and measure. But really, the unseen is often more powerful than the visible. We've been conditioned to believe in separation, that we are isolated individuals in a fragmented world, yet in truth, we are inseparable from the oneness of the Field. We are intricately connected to all that exists.

You might think, 'Wait, aren't you talking about God, the Source, the Universe?'. Many terms describe this profound, universal energy, but all refer to the same all-powerful, interconnected energy that is the creator of everything. While this force needs no words, we turn to language to understand our place in the world. Despite our best efforts, capturing this force in words is impossible, as our language can not do it justice.

Varied cultures, philosophies and spiritual practices teach the Field. Each reflects a unique perspective, but ultimately, they speak the same truth. Whether you see it from a scientific, spiritual or religious perspective, this universal connection is the foundation of everything.

A Universal Connection

Before we dive into the science and relationship we have with the Field, we will look at where it fits in the minds of society. Many people who start on a spiritual awakening or self-exploration may wonder where their religion fits into this journey. They might face judgment from people in their lives who view spirituality and religion as opposing forces. What if there's no separation? What if they're just different ways of connecting to the same universal truth? This apparent opposition makes us ask the question - Does the Field counter religion? My take is that no, it explains religion because it is the science behind spirituality. There is nothing that is not part of the Field; therefore, there is nothing that is not God and pure love.

Imagine a world where all religions are united, each seen as a different expression of the same universal truth. A world without fighting or judgment, where people honour one another's beliefs as paths to the same shared source. What if these diverse perspectives brought us closer instead of dividing us and showed us the many faces of love, compassion, and connection? This vision isn't about blending beliefs, but embracing the common thread that links us all. Because the quality of this force is indescribable, problems may arise when individuals consider their perception as the only truth.

Let's look at how various faiths describe the universal connection (the Field).

1. **Buddhism:** In Buddhism, the interconnectedness of all things is central. They believe everything is interconnected, like a giant web. Buddhist beliefs sometimes describe Dharmakaya as a formless energy field that fills all of existence.

2. **Christianity**: In Christianity, the Holy Spirit is an invisible but ever-present divine force that connects us to God and each other. Some Christians see this as an omnipresent energy of love and grace through which one can experience a sense of oneness with the divine.

3. **Hinduism:** Hindu teachings describe Brahman as the ultimate, formless reality that underlies everything. Brahman is an all-pervading force within and around us, often described as an infinite cosmic consciousness. Prana, or life energy, is also significant and described as a force flowing through everything.

4. **Taoism:** The Tao, or Way, is the natural force underlying existence, the source of all creation and the guiding principle of life. This resonates with the idea of a unifying field that connects and guides everything in the universe.

5. **Islam:** In Sufi mysticism, God is an all-encompassing presence, often described as *Al-Haqq* (the Truth) or *Al-Wadud* (the Loving). For Sufis, God's oneness is reflected in all existence, a unity frequently felt through mystical experience.

6. **Judaism:** In Kabbalah, the mystical branch of Judaism, there is the concept of *Ein Sof* (the Infinite). Ein Sof represents God's boundless, indescribable essence, present everywhere and beyond time and space. This energy flows into the world, connecting everything as a continuous, divine presence.

These descriptions all sound the same, right? I think of it this way: imagine a group of people describing the same breathtaking mountain, but each from a different side. One sees rolling meadows, another marvels at rocky cliffs, while another is captivated by cascading waterfalls. They're all describing the same mountain, just from their unique perspective. Religion and spirituality work the same way — different views, one shared truth.

Unfortunately, throughout our world, religion has become polarised and divisive. What I have always found interesting is that what connects us all is what can cause division. Really though, there's a profound beauty in honouring the diversity of beliefs while recognising the common ground that binds us all. Looking at the big picture, we all originate from innocent beginnings and love. We are all born knowing we are part of oneness, but we have unlearnt this. We talk about this unlearning again throughout the book. My thoughts are this: a religion or spirituality that inspires fear, judgement, and restriction isn't helpful. True faith should bring love, infiniteness, unconditional love and joy. If that is what you are experiencing, you're on the right path. OK, I digress, but open discussion and respect for opinions help you expand your awareness. Let's discuss why people see the Field so differently – yet the same.

~

As you can see, describing the Field can be confusing because of all the different words and beliefs. This chapter has been the most challenging to write, and many pages have been sent to the shredder to try and keep this simple. How do you describe something that doesn't fit in our language? I'm sure it would resonate instantly if I could send you telepathic energy waves. Descriptions of the Field seem to merge but also conflict, leaving us wondering how all these perspectives can coexist. Neither perspective is wrong, and they can even overlap.

I have made sense of this in my mind by a fascinating principle in quantum physics called the observer effect, which shows that the act of observation influences what is being observed. Studies have shown that tiny particles, like electrons, behave like waves of possibilities when not being observed. But when someone observes them, they 'collapse' into a specific location or state, behaving like a particle. Some describe the observer effect as more straightforward: imagine a tree falling in the forest. Does it make a sound if no one is there to hear it? While sound waves may exist, the experience of sound requires an observer. This simple explanation highlights how observation shapes reality, much like how everyone experiences and describes the Field differently. The Field seems to shape itself to meet us where we are, reflecting what we need or are ready to see. It expresses itself depending on what resonates most with each person's beliefs, cultural background, or spiritual understanding. This expression allows us to connect with it on a personal level.

Throughout this book, I have taken the middle ground on some heavy topics, coming from a neutral territory. However we experience it, the Field is an energy of love that creates everything. These descriptions are my understanding of the Field, and I remain open to learning and seeing things differently as new ideas emerge.

The good news is that when you know there's more to you than your physical body, your perspective changes, no matter your beliefs. This faith opens you to a deeper connection with love and energy through prayer, meditation, or simply being present (yes, even while waiting in line for coffee). The Field is always available, and you can rely on it, like Wi-Fi — no, it's much more reliable than Wi-Fi. The Field is always there, no matter what. By the end of this book, you should feel much closer to the Field and have all the skills to utilise its unlimited gifts.

Whatever your beliefs, science tells us there is a unified force. As scientists delve deeper into quantum physics, they uncover more about this force. It's almost as though the universe is winking at us, saying, 'You're all getting warmer'.

Breaking Down the Dense Science

Let's back up and talk science. I'm no scientist, and honestly, it's not my passion, but I know some of you need hard proof before moving into the 'knowing.' Okay, let's break it down because understanding the science at a very basic level will help solidify your belief that the Field is accessible to you. Did you know we are mainly energy? Science tells us that everything, including our bodies, is made up of atoms, and here's the fascinating part: about 99% of each atom is space, or what scientists now describe as energy fields. Even more incredible is that these energy fields aren't static (meaning still or stationary); they're dynamic, constantly shifting and exchanging information with the world around them. Imagine it like a field of tall grass. A single breeze sends waves rippling through the blades, each influencing the movements of those around it. This constant interaction mirrors how energy fields shift and exchange information, connecting everything around us. This dynamic flow of energy is why the Field can influence us so profoundly; we are energy, and the Field is energy.

To understand how all this works, we need to zoom in on the type of science that studies these energy fields. Enter quantum science. While mainstream science focuses on big, predictable interactions, quantum science dives into the smallest particles and their strange, interconnected behaviours. Let's break down the difference between the two sciences with a simple analogy. Imagine you have a camera with two zoom settings, a wide-angle lens and a microscope. Mainstream science is like the wide-angle lens; it looks at the big picture, studying larger objects and their predictable, clockwork-like interactions. Quantum science, on the other hand, is like using a microscope. It zooms in on the tiniest particles, uncovering their bizarre and interconnected behaviours. Without quantum science, we wouldn't have the tools to explore or explain the unseen force we call the Field.

And now, here is a little history of these two sciences. In the late 17th century, Sir Isaac Newton revolutionised our understanding of the world. His theories painted the universe as a giant, predictable machine, with everything operating separately in neat little compartments. This view was groundbreaking for its time and still dominates many scientific circles today. Newton's framework works brilliantly for explaining larger, everyday phenomena, like the motion of planets or why apples fall from trees. However, it struggles when we try to understand the messy, interconnected nature of life and the universe.

Then came quantum physics. It began to take shape in the early 20th century, thanks to trailblazers like Albert Einstein and Niels Bohr. They proposed something radical: that reality isn't as separate as it seems. Instead, it's deeply interconnected at its core. These discoveries flipped the script, shifting science from a mechanical view of the universe to one that recognised a web of connections (the Field). For the first time, science started to align with ancient philosophies, blending ideas of oneness and interconnectedness in ways that would've made Newton raise an eyebrow.

Fast forward to today. Quantum physics isn't just mainstream—it's becoming inseparable from modern science, taught in universities around the globe. Quantum discoveries have revealed particles that defy logic, ignore distance, and behave in ways that make you seriously question reality itself. It has shown that the Field has an innate intelligent consciousness. Once dismissed as fringe theories, these ideas are now reshaping how we understand the universe. It's no wonder that ancient philosophies and modern theories often converge on the idea that something greater may be at play.

While the details can get wildly complex, the core concepts are nothing short of fascinating. Take quantum entanglement, for example, where two particles become so intertwined that whatever happens to one instantly affects the other, even if they're galaxies apart. Think of them as cosmic BFFs, connected no matter the distance. I'll dive into that next — it's truly mind-blowing.

Let's talk about quantum entanglement in a way that makes sense in everyday life. Entanglement is basically when two particles are in contact and then separated by a vast distance but are still connected. Imagine you and your best friend each take a matching pair of enchanted walkie-talkies. One of you heads to New York, the other to Tokyo. Here's the weird part: no matter how far apart you are, if one of you presses the button, the other walkie-talkie instantly lights up. No lag, no delay. It's as if the two walkie-talkies are having their own secret conversation across the globe. We can compare quantum entanglement to the deep connection people sometimes feel with others, even across great distances or beyond this physical world. For instance, some twins report sensing each other's emotions or experiences, no matter how far apart they are. In the physical realm, quantum entanglement shows how particles can remain linked and respond to each other instantly, no matter the space or distance between them. Some believe quantum entanglement could explain telepathy, suggesting that minds, like entangled particles, may stay connected no matter the distance. Quantum entanglement is very real, and in 2022, the Nobel Prize in Physics was awarded jointly to three physicists for their studies on quantum entanglement.

So, if quantum entanglement is when two particles become so interconnected that they communicate instantly, even if separated by vast distances, how does it work? Scientists do not know exactly how this works. (Spoiler: it might involve the Field).

I wrote this book to give you a foundational understanding of concepts like the Field without delving too deeply into its science. I hope I have offered you an explanation of the basics. For me, I know that once I felt it, really felt it, I no longer needed to know the exact science. For those interested in exploring detailed science, I encourage you to dive into the works of leaders in this space, like Gregg Braden or Lynne McTaggart.

Two of my favourite teachers in the quantum field space today are:

- **Dr Joe Dispenza** – He combines neuroscience, psychoneuroimmunology (*whoa, big word; it's the study of how your thoughts, emotions and brain influence your immune system and overall health*), epigenetics and quantum physics. This blend teaches people how their thoughts and feelings impact their biology and reality. In his books and retreats, he teaches people to tap into the Field for healing and transformation and to create the life they desire.

- **Bruce H Lipton, Ph.D.** Bruce has gained recognition for his work on epigenetics and the idea that consciousness and beliefs directly influence our biology. Lipton highlights the subconscious mind's ability to influence our genes and health via the Field. We will discuss epigenetics later on in the book.

There are, of course, many more amazing teachers bridging science with spirituality. They help us understand mystical concepts that once seemed woo-woo to some. Actually, those way outside *Opposite World* probably still think it's woo-woo. But please note that I'm not here to teach you anyone's work; instead, I'll share my experiences and understandings.

The Field Is Like a Boomerang

The Field isn't random; it follows a special rule called 'like attracts like'. You have probably heard of the law of attraction. The law of attraction means that the energy we send out into the Field attracts similar energy back to us. Like the internet has algorithms and keeps showing you what you focus on, the Field will show you more of what you think and feel. Basically, your external world is a manifestation of your inner dialogue. So essentially, as you will begin to discover throughout this guide, change your thoughts and feelings (your energy), and you'll change your life.

It's sometimes easier to understand things by observing people; think about the people you know. We've all met that person who's always complaining about something. For them, nothing ever goes right —every restaurant messes up their order, every event is a disaster, traffic is always too slow (or too fast) and somehow, every relationship turns into a soap opera. Even the grocery store assistant can't pack their bags properly — because, of course, the bread ends up squashed under the canned goods. It's almost like drama has them on speed dial. Why? Because they've built a field around them, a neon sign saying, 'Chaos welcome!'. This constant energy of stress and negativity keeps them stuck in a loop of 'Why me?' moments, attracting more of the same. The Field, ever-magnetic, simply mirrors their frequency — delivering exactly what they're broadcasting.

Now, think about someone who radiates positivity, the friend who seems like they've won the cosmic lottery. They're joyful, kind, optimistic, and probably the person who somehow befriends every dog in the park. People always tell them they're lucky or blessed, but the truth is, they're just vibing at a higher frequency.

Now, you might wonder, if the Field, at its core, is unconditional love, why doesn't it shower us all with only good vibes? Here's the thing — the Field is neutral. It doesn't know good from bad; it simply reflects the energy we send out, like a cosmic mirror. The Field doesn't judge; it just is. This neutrality gives us the freedom to create, learn, and grow, but it also means we must take responsibility for the energy we contribute.

As you work through the book, please remember that our thoughts, beliefs and emotions come back to us as our experiences; it is essential to know this. It's crucial you don't just have knowledge of this but also understand the wisdom and live by it.

You can do some amazing things once you tap into the field and learn how to shift your frequency. You will begin to heal, transform and become the master in your life. Let's keep exploring how vast this Field really is.

Planetary Connections

Not only does the Field connect to us, but it also connects us with the planets, the moon, and the sun, aligning us with the rhythms of creation. People have long believed that the moon and planets subtly influence our moods, emotions, and even life events because of our alignment with the Field. Think about this: the moon, with its gravitational pull, affects tides and water flow on Earth. Since our bodies are primarily water, this lunar energy profoundly impacts us, particularly during a full moon, which often brings heightened emotions and clarity, helping us identify what we need to release. I have worked in a hospital as a nurse and can confirm the emotional difference of patients on a full moon. Females often say that their menstrual cycle aligns with the moon or even with other females they spend a lot of time with. OK, I'll backtrack here so you don't think I'm crazy. I just said our bodies are primarily water, but earlier, I told you our bodies are 99% energy. Let me explain that. We're also mostly water because water is energy. At the atomic level, water is made of vibrating particles, and like everything else, it's 99% empty space filled with energy.

A remarkable example of our interconnectedness is how animals and plants sense their humans, regardless of the distance. For instance, studies have suggested that plants can detect their owner's presence up to two kilometres away. Similarly, many pet owners, myself included, can attest to the uncanny ability of dogs to 'know' when their humans are coming home. Take my dogs, for instance; they rush to the door in excitement as one of us nears, even before the car is in sight. Our family has observed this for years, but just recently, I learned that there is a book about this phenomenon called Dogs That Know When Their Owners Are Coming Home: And Other Unexplained Powers of Animals by Rupert Sheldrake. This phenomenon beautifully shows that these invisible threads connecting us to the Field extend to all living beings.

Have You Felt It?

I'll give examples of how the Field can be noticed in your *daily life*. *Has* someone suddenly come to mind after a long time? Perhaps a friend or foe, and then you unexpectedly see them soon after. Or what about when you stand in nature and feel a deep sense of belonging? These moments may feel fleeting, but they are glimpses into something profound, the unseen force that binds us all. While these are subtle experiences, those who regularly meditate, practice energy healing or work with intuitive states often feel the Field in a much more tangible, undeniable way.

Let's try a little experiment to show you how you can feel energy. Rub your palms together briskly for a few seconds, then drag them slowly, holding them a few inches apart. Notice the tingling, warmth or gentle pressure between your hands? That's energy. What you feel is your body's natural energy at work, a small glimpse of the powerful forces that constantly flow through and around us. This energy isn't isolated to just your hands; it's connected to everything around you, part of the invisible Field that links all life.

I usually feel the divine Field of energy the strongest when in group meditations. I used to think it was a little strange, all these people meditating together. I considered meditation a private activity until I first felt its potency. Being in that shared space and feeling everyone's energy align was like tapping into something bigger than myself. Once you experience that, everything you thought you knew about connection changes. I will describe how it feels when I am connected and focusing on the Field. Remember, though, that everyone feels it differently. Here is my description: Imagine the feeling of being in a warm bath, gently moving your arms through the water. You can sense the soft yet firm pressure of the water against your skin. Now, picture that this water doesn't just surround you; it penetrates your skin and envelops every cell in your body. The density or pressure feels like water, but the material feels electrical. This sensation is light and powerful, a tingling, electric energy flowing through you. And within this energy lies the most profound sense of love you've ever experienced, a love so pure and encompassing it defies words.

It's not just in deep meditation that you can feel the Field; you've likely experienced it in everyday moments. Think about a time when you walked into a room and instantly sensed tension or unease, even before anyone spoke. That immediate feeling isn't just intuition — it's your ability to pick up on different frequencies within the Field. Everything carries a frequency, from people to objects to the spaces we inhabit. These energetic imprints can linger long after the person or event has passed. These imprints could explain why some places feel warm and inviting while others feel heavy or unsettling. Over time, as you become more attuned to this invisible field, you may start to notice these subtle energies more clearly.

So, just as each person radiates their unique energetic signature, objects can hold on to the lingering frequency of past events or people. This imprint is why letting go of objects that no longer serve you can be so powerful—you might unknowingly be holding on to low-frequency energy, whether from your past or someone else's. Think about a toxic breakup where one person leaves behind their belongings; that energy remains. Clearing out these objects can help shift the energy in your space. On the flip side, you might have an item that carries a beautiful, high-frequency energy — something infused with love, joy, or meaning — so you naturally want to keep it close.

As I was writing this, I had a memory pop up out of nowhere. It ties in with low-frequency emotions lingering in a location. I once visited a beer brewery in Byron Bay, and as soon as I stepped into a large conference room, I felt an instant wave of negative energy. This energy felt so overwhelming that I almost ran out. Actually, the truth is, I did run out and may have let out a small scream. At that time, I didn't know much about energy; my first thought was that the room may be haunted. I even asked the barman if the room was ghostly, but he said nothing. Later, the owner approached me and asked me to point out where I felt that strange energy. He told me the exact spot was atop an old pig slaughterhouse.

How Can I Tap into the Field?

You don't have to have secret skills to tap into this energy. It's right here for all of us, wrapped around and within us, no matter who we are or our past. Let this be your reminder that you're never alone in this journey.

To tune into the Field, we must first align our energies with its higher frequency. Stop now, find quiet and stillness, and get out of your mind. You may sense it. To connect on a deep level, we may need to dissolve aspects within us that don't have a frequency match with the Field. In this book, we call these shadows, which act as barriers between us and the Field. We will work on these later to tune into the Field fully.

Could Children Learn to Tap into the Field?

I've always been passionate about teaching children about their innate abilities, which are not typically covered in school. Understanding these concepts helps them build resilience and strength when facing life's challenges. The language in this book is simple enough for curious teenagers and even younger readers. It would be a gift for them to learn this at such a confusing age!

Kids today grow up in a constantly connected world where technology and social media offer both opportunities and pressures. The pressures make it easy for them to feel overwhelmed, lost, and perhaps alone. The Field and other strategies in the book could offer them a path to something more meaningful than social media or fleeting trends. Knowing that their thoughts, actions, and emotions will create the energy that shapes their experiences could positively impact their lives. This shift in mindset can offer children a more empowering way to live, steering them away from the prevalent victim mindset. When children or even young adults realise they're part of this powerful, interconnected field, they gain a sense of purpose and control. This knowledge will teach them to be positive, have good relationships, foster mental wellness and cope with stress. Recognising the power they hold within themselves can be incredibly empowering.

The younger humans are, the closer they are to the Field, as they haven't been as heavily programmed by society and still have greater access to the creative parts of their brain. Societal expectations and school pressures have yet to take over their left analytical mind.

This knowledge can be a guiding tool, helping children make choices that align with their true selves and what they wish to create in their lives. Imagine a generation of self-aware, compassionate kids who can manage their emotions.

Children could find peace in solitude and stillness instead of getting caught up in the distractions of the matrix. This internal peace would be my wish for future generations.

~

The Field sounds like magic, doesn't it? No wonder we're so obsessed with superheroes and magic movies. Why do you think that is? Deep down, we know we have powers; we've simply forgotten how to use them. Now, envision utilising this power to craft your heaven on earth; it isn't just a dream — it's entirely possible. We will continue to connect to the field throughout the book, and in Chapter 7, we will discuss how it relates to our bodies, awareness, and dimensions.

By the end of this book, I hope you'll find tuning into the Field as easy as changing the channel on your television. While we may not be able to access the Field immediately, our journey of inner understanding will guide us there, one step at a time. Our bridge won't be a direct route; there may be obstacles to clear on the way, but together, we will turn the process into a fun adventure.

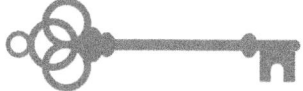

You are always connected — trust and tune in.

Important Note About the Bridge
You'll often hear me refer to a bridge when connecting to the Field. Let me clarify something important: you're not reaching for or travelling to the Field as if it's somewhere outside you. You're already connected to it, you are it. It's an inseparable part of who you are. However, obstacles or blocks may cloud your awareness of this connection, making it feel out of reach. The bridge is simply a metaphor for clearing those barriers and consciously rediscovering what's always there. It's not about seeking — it's about remembering.

CHAPTER 2

A RESILIENT HEART

Heart Coherence

As we delved into the concept of the Field, we uncovered the profound truth that our inner state directly shapes our external reality. We will now discover the transformative power of heart coherence. What is coherence? Picture a synchronised marching band or a team of synchronised swimmers moving as one, their efforts merging into a unified whole. Heart coherence is much the same; the harmonious alignment of our heart, mind and emotions creates a state of flow that resonates with the energy of the Field. Heart coherence is the heart of this book, literally and metaphorically, because the heart is the foundation, the glue that binds everything we'll explore. Coherence unlocks our potential to connect deeply and transform ourselves and the world.

To understand heart coherence, let's first explore its opposite: heart incoherence. Your heart becomes incoherent when your body is stuck in stress mode, and your heart and brain are entirely out of sync. Think of it as two people trying to row a boat in opposite directions. When you're overwhelmed by negative emotions like fear, guilt, anger or anxiety, your body goes into overdrive. Unfortunately, many of us live in this state so often that it's like stress has unpacked its bags and made itself at home. Sound familiar?

When your heart is incoherent, its rhythms become jagged and irregular. Your poor heart is trying to beat against a closed system as it whispers, 'It's not safe to open', pulling back to protect itself. As the heart pulls back, it can create a barrier that leaves the person feeling isolated and disconnected from themselves and others. Why does this happen? Because your body has gone into fight-or-flight mode, that ancient survival system meant for emergencies like running from a predator. Our body's fight-or-flight response is meant to be a short-term survival mechanism, yet many people today remain in constant stress. This constant stress mode makes people feel like they are swimming upstream with a backpack full of rocks. Internal chaos disrupts communication between the heart and brain, causing stress and depleting energy. The brain becomes hyper-alert, and everything feels like a crisis. It's like living in high-definition drama mode. Their focus narrows, tunnel vision sets in, and it feels impossible to see beyond their current state. Understanding this inner turmoil can help you be more self-aware and allow compassion for others facing stress. For someone in a calm, coherent state, this incoherent energy in others can feel like a whirlwind of chaos; it's exhausting to be around. But the good news? By choosing heart coherence, you can shift your energy and create a ripple effect in the world around you.

What physically happens to your body in this fight-or-flight mode? Your body shifts into survival mode, sending blood to your arms and legs so you can run or fight. Meanwhile, your body pauses your digestive and immune systems and other bodily functions. It's like your body says, 'We'll deal with digestion later; right now, we must escape the imaginary tiger!'. Our bodies are not supposed to be in this state for a prolonged period. When stress causes people's hearts to hide and their bodies to slow or pause natural bodily systems, declining health is inevitable. It's hard to thrive when your body thinks it's constantly fighting for survival. I think you get my point on why we need to manage our emotions and live through our hearts.

The Heart Is the Real Boss

When we step out of the stress response and embrace positive emotions like gratitude, love, or peace, something remarkable happens: Our heart rhythms become smooth and harmonious. This state, known as heart coherence, acts like a master conductor, bringing the body into a state of balance. Brain function improves, hormones find their rhythm, and a sense of well-being flows. Imagine a stone dropped into calm water, sending gentle, synchronised ripples. That's the wave you want to create around your heart.

This book shows how to overcome lasting negative emotional states. But if you're in an acute situation and want to rise above it, try shifting your focus to your heart. Where focus goes, energy flows. Directing energy to your heart helps it find a smooth, harmonious rhythm, creating a beautiful, coherent field around it.

Once your heart reaches a coherent state, it sends a message to the brain: 'Hey, we're safe now. It's time to switch off the alarm bells.' This gentle signal pulls the brain out of panic mode and ushers it into a more creative, relaxed state. Suddenly, the brain perks up, like a performer reassured that the stage is set. The brain fog clears, clarity returns, and problem-solving becomes possible again.

Here's something you may not have heard. It's not the brain that runs the show; it's the heart that is in charge. So, what is the brain's role? It's like the assistant who writes everything down, nods knowingly, and tries to look important. The heart is the boss — always has been. Research shows that the heart sends more signals to the brain than the brain sends to the heart. The heart communicates through four key pathways: neurological (via the vagus nerve), biochemical (hormones like oxytocin), biophysical (pulse waves), and energetic (electromagnetic fields). Another interesting fact is that the heart even has its own neuronal network of about 40,000 neurons; this is why it is sometimes called the 'heart brain,' allowing it to process information independently. Studies from the HeartMath Institute show that when the heart is in a coherent rhythm (triggered by gratitude, love, or deep breathing), it will optimise brain function, enhance emotional balance, and even improve decision-making.

In contrast, erratic heart rhythms caused by stress or frustration disrupt this flow, impacting cognitive clarity. Essentially, the heart is not just pumping blood; it's shaping your reality. That's why a coherent heart naturally leads to a coherent brain. When the heart takes the lead, everything else falls into place.

A calm heart provides strength, resilience and peace to overcome life's storms. A coherent heart isn't just about bouncing back from current challenges; it's about having the resilience to take on any of life's future chaos. This state doesn't just uplift your emotions and mindset; it also positively affects your physical health. A coherent heart promotes better circulation, reduces stress on the body, and supports overall well-being. We'll explore the connection between your emotional state and health later in the book. One of my favourite mantras is 'What would love do?'. When making decisions or facing problems, focus on your heart and tackle whatever it is from there.

Coherence as a Collective

In addition to heart coherence's mental and physical aspects, we can enhance our ability to tune into the Field with clarity and intention. Remember from the last chapter that we are energy, constantly projecting our frequencies into the Field. When we are in heart coherence, the frequency we emit is high, like love. This high frequency, in turn, can help bring coherence to the Fields of others, whether they are physically near us or far away but connected to our intentions. Later in the book, we'll explore studies demonstrating the power of groups entering heart coherence together during meditation. I've experienced this firsthand as I participate in distance coherent healing regularly. Group consciousness holds incredible power and coherence, and incoherence significantly influences the Field. Want to hear proof of this? There is a machine called a REG (random event generator), which measures fluctuations in collective consciousness. Studies during significant global events such as 9/11 and the death of

Princess Diana showed measurable shifts in the machine's readings. These examples highlight how collective emotional states can impact the Field, whether coherent, such as during moments of love and unity, or incoherent, like during fear and chaos. These findings support the idea that achieving a state of unified heart coherence and emotional harmony strengthens our connection to the Field, creating a ripple effect that influences the collective consciousness. So come on, you owe it to humanity to be in heart coherence and do your bit for the Field that surrounds us all. I sometimes play with this in public and focus on transmuting frequency in places I feel could benefit.

Grasping science concepts like the REG machine can help you comprehend how such a thing is possible. Let's get a little bit more sciencey.

What Science Says

From a scientific perspective, energy waves, whether sound, light, or electromagnetic waves, need order or coherence to function effectively. On the flip side, when waves are out of sync or chaotic, they interfere with each other, cancelling out their potential energy. This destructive interference reduces their effectiveness and creates disorder. Remember, we are mostly energy, and you don't want this disorder going on with your heart.

Remember this: Your heart is more than just a muscle pumping blood. It's the centre of your emotional and energetic well-being, radiating signals to every cell in your body and extending far beyond it. I'll explain more about that shortly.

Not only does the heart radiate signals to every cell — it goes much further. Scientists say the heart produces the human body's most powerful electromagnetic field. The heart's energy is measurable several feet away, and the energy changes with your emotional state. The HeartMath Institute has shown that the heart's electromagnetic field affects the body and can transmit emotions between people.

As shown above, you measure the energy produced by your heart externally, but you can also measure your heart coherence internally. How? Through heart rate variability analysis (HRV). HRV assesses the variations in time intervals between heartbeats. A coherent heart rhythm exhibits a stable, regular, and repeating pattern, often resembling a sine wave at a single frequency. This stability results in a higher score.

But beyond the measurable lies something even more incredible. The heart is the gateway to love, the highest frequency of all. Love is our end goal; it's the key to everything. Love isn't just an emotion; it's the energy that connects us to ourselves, others, and the *Field* and opens us to infinite possibilities. A coherent heart radiates a strong field that can dissolve boundaries, inspire kindness, and transform the world around you. Love, at its core, is everything, and the energy of the heart is the beacon that guides us back to it. A coherent heart helps you bounce back from challenges; this resilience allows you to stay grounded in love no matter what life throws your way.

If you are feeling any stress, a great tool you can have 'on call' is to stop and breathe through your heart. We will discuss that a little more shortly.

Live Through Your Heart

I want to introduce you to Jane, a self-proclaimed stress magnet. Her days were a whirlwind of little disasters: coffee spills, endless traffic, and mysteriously disappeared emails. One day, after a chaotic morning capped off by her toddler painting the couch with yogurt, Jane realised something had to change. She wanted to get a grip on her emotions. Her body was feeling the toll, with constant headaches, heart palpitations, tight shoulders, and poor sleep.

That evening, she came across an article about managing stress. It discussed a breathing technique and how to elevate her emotions. 'It's worth a try,' she thought.

The next time life threw Jane a curveball (a forgotten lunch meeting), she paused, closed her eyes, and started her box breathing. She went for it, in… two… three… four… hold… two… three… four… Jane paired each breath with thoughts of gratitude — how her coworker offered to share their sandwich and how her child's laughter made the yogurt mess almost worth it. To her surprise, she felt calmer, lighter, and less rattled. It felt like an internal reset.

After a few weeks, her smartwatch, which tracked her heart rate variability (HRV), confirmed the difference. Her HRV readings had always hovered around 25 — low and indicative of stress. But as she continued combining box breathing with gratitude and love, her HRV climbed steadily to 45, showing her nervous system was finding balance. Her heart had now gone from being incoherent to coherent.

Jane's minor health issues and heart palpitations began to fade. Her headaches became rare, her shoulders relaxed, and she even started sleeping through the night. Over the next few weeks, this combination of breathing and emotional elevation became her secret weapon. She wasn't a stress magnet anymore; she was the calm amidst the storm, radiating joy and gratitude.

But Jane knew this was just the beginning. She realised she needed to address the root causes of her stress — her negative mindset and buried emotions. Now that her brain was no longer consumed with constant chatter and she felt less stressed, she was ready to tackle the steps in *Opposite World*.

~

Heart Breathing Exercise: In the last chapter, we did a little exercise, feeling the surrounding energy; now, let us do one to feel through our hearts. Sit quietly and breathe in and out of your chest area. Putting your awareness in the region creates energy. Now relax into your heart and stay there. On a slow inhalation, imagine breathing in divine love and on the exhalation, radiate gratitude. Breathe in love and out gratitude. In with love: Out with gratitude…keep going. Doing this elevates your spirit and helps to bring your heart, mind, emotions and body into coherent alignment and stillness. Do this often in your day to create the frequency of love within and around you. Make time during the day to open your heart. Try to elevate your emotions to love, even if you're having a bad day. Focus on something you are grateful for or love, and sit with that. You can do heart breathing anywhere — in your car, on a break at work, on a walk or at the grocery store. It's a simple practice but can be very effective. Why is it so important to do this when feeling stressed? Because when you're deeply focused on heart coherence and generating feelings of love, gratitude, or appreciation, it becomes difficult — if not impossible — to simultaneously feel negative emotions like fear, anger, or anxiety. Think of it like this: You can't simultaneously tune in to two radio stations from one device.

The world would be beautiful if everyone resonated with this love frequency. Envision a world filled with open hearts, compassion, and joy in every person. We are all part of the ripple, so do your part and open your heart when you are out and about; you never know who it may affect or even heal.

If you would like to learn more about heart coherence and the science backing it, the HeartMath Institute has a lot of information on its website. They also offer apps and other technology to measure your heart's coherence.

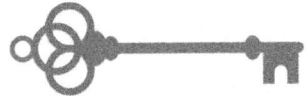

Live through the heart.

CHAPTER 3

WHO AM I?

STEP 1

Self-Discovery

The Mirror Within

Self-reflection — truly understand yourself.

As explained in the previous chapters, the Field isn't just some mystical force hanging out in the cosmos; it's like the universe's Snapchat filter, constantly reflecting what's happening inside us. The Field doesn't just take some of your thoughts and emotions and disregard others; it matches the frequencies of everything.

Before diving into the exciting realms of meditation and creating your desired life, we will take some time for self-exploration. Who are you at your core? What are the beliefs, values, and desires that define you? Which areas of your life are not stacking up? What do you truly want, not what others want of you — what do YOU want? Only by understanding and aligning with our authentic selves can we unlock our full potential and the magic of the Field.

In this chapter, you will discover how and why you need to know yourself and your true essence. Try to think of the Field as a mirror; it reveals how our thoughts, emotions and beliefs shape the reality we experience. Feeling Zen? The world around you might sparkle. Feeling like a hot mess? Expect life to resemble a soap opera. When we understand this connection, we see that our world is not separate but intricately linked to our inner state. So many people are unaware that the life they are living is a mirror of their emotions, thoughts and beliefs. It's a challenging concept for people to get their heads around. Why is it so hard? Because we have to turn around and look at ourselves; it's so much easier to be a victim in the world or resign ourselves to the belief that this is just the life we've been dealt with. In the following four chapters, we will go through four steps to help get to know ourselves deeper, pay attention to our thoughts, and manage our emotions. These four steps will help clear our bridge to our true selves and the Field. To create change, you must be the master of your life, the expert of you.

We spend so much time analysing and judging the people we meet, especially those who catch our attention in relationships. When someone new enters our orbit, we morph into amateur detectives, scrutinising their every move. *Who is this person? What are their strengths, flaws, and secrets hidden beneath the surface?* We probe their characters like an audition for a role or a job interview, searching for light and shadow to decide if they're worth a spot in our lives.

Enter *Opposite World*, where the script flips. How often do we turn that same magnifying glass inward? Why do we pour so much energy into dissecting others while we give ourselves just a passing glance in the mirror? Imagine if we treated our quirks, strengths, and flaws with the same level of fascination. What might we discover? It's funny how we can spot the tiniest speck of dust on someone else's mirror but somehow miss the cracks in our own.

The truth is that the people we choose to keep close, especially in romantic relationships, are often our mirror. They reflect parts of us that we may not have acknowledged. Sometimes, it's flattering, like seeing our best qualities highlighted. Other times, it's like catching a glimpse of ourselves in bad lighting; it's uncomfortable, but it's still us. These relationships reveal truths about our strengths and, more importantly, our shadows. Until we take the time to explore these shadows or emotional blocks, we might find part of our life stuck in an endless loop to nowhere. We may continue to be drawn to the same kinds of people, wondering why we're stuck in a rerun of the same old relationship drama. (Spoiler alert: it's not just them — it's us, too.) How often do we hear people blame others for their problems? *'I always pick the wrong guys/girls'* - *'All the women I hang out with are bitches'* - *'Everyone in my life is judgmental'* - *'Every time I go out for lunch, I get rude staff who always make mistakes'*. Instead, they should be saying, why am I attracting groups of people with the same traits? Maybe you are a giant magnet.

Here is a typical example: Meet Asha; she keeps dating the same type of guy: emotionally unavailable and distant. Instead of blaming the world, she stops to pause and reflect. *Could this pattern be the mirror of my fear of vulnerability and self-doubt?* When she began working on her inner beliefs and energy, the Field started reflecting a different reality. Doing a small amount of self-reflection offers Asha a new reality, and she plans to get to the bottom of where those fears even came from.

As you read this chapter, I invite you to consider how your relationships, both past and present, have served as mirrors, offering glimpses into your beautiful soul. Perhaps, by turning that mirror inward, you'll find a deeper connection with yourself and those around you. Remember, while self-reflection and getting to know yourself better are essential, it's not about 'fixing' yourself. Where you are today and who you are is perfect for this moment in your timeline, even if the reasons aren't entirely clear. And where will you be tomorrow? That will be shaped by your choices, opening doors to new timelines and possibilities.

So, flip the script and start paying attention to the people in your life for who they are and what they might teach you about yourself. I invite you to take quiet moments to reflect, be mindful, and observe your thoughts and feelings. If writing is your thing, write in a journal about what makes you happy, what triggers you, and what these moments reveal about your inner world. Look beyond your reflection in the mirror and delve into the captivating individual staring back at you. Why? Self-discovery is one of the key ways to enter *Opposite World*.

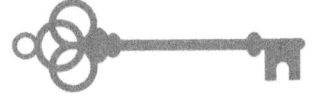

I see myself in the reflection of others.

Self-Reflection

In the last section, we explored how the people in our lives can act as mirrors, revealing aspects of ourselves we may not always see. It's not just people in our lives that act as a reflection of ourselves, but every aspect of our life — our job, environment, habits, possessions, and even the challenges we face. They all mirror aspects of who we are and what we believe. We can understand ourselves more deeply by paying attention to these reflections. Self-discovery doesn't stop with your internal senses. Many tools and approaches help us get to know ourselves a little better. We don't only have to focus on our deep inner world; we can also get to know our personalities. Are you intrigued by your personality or your soul's wishes? Check out these fun options:

1. **Gene Keys** (Richard Rudd): A contemplative system that uses your astrological chart to help you unlock your highest potential. Each key unlocks different parts of you, revealing talents and challenges to help you grow. Richard's work is fascinating, offering incredible depth to those ready to explore. I only recently realised that writing this book aligns perfectly with my Life's Work Gene Key. According to my key, my purpose is transforming limiting thoughts and old patterns into new perspectives and enlightenment. As I wrote each chapter, I found myself doing just that — challenging old ways of thinking, exploring new ideas, and helping others see beyond their limitations. I always feel the most satisfied when I can help people transmute their thoughts and see life differently. This realisation made me appreciate the Gene Keys even more, as it showed me that I'm living my purpose through writing this book. It's a powerful reminder that we're often guided to our

true path without realising it. The key is to watch how you feel when you do things.

If you're curious to explore your purpose or understand why specific challenges or gifts keep showing up, I highly recommend diving into the Gene Keys. Who knows, you might discover that you're already living your purpose, too.

2. **Astrology**: Birth chart astrology illuminates life paths and personal struggles.
3. **Myers-Briggs Type Indicator** (MBTI): The MBTI personality test helps you understand your decision-making style and how you relate to others. Many corporate professionals study this work.
4. **Love Languages** (Gary Chapman): This is an oldy but a goody, so powerful. This book identifies five primary ways people express and receive love: through words of affirmation, acts of service, gifts, quality time, or physical touch. Knowing one's love language can deepen relationships and enhance self-understanding. Relationships benefit from this handy, simple tool.
5. **Human Design**: By blending several ancient and modern systems, human design provides a blueprint for how energy flows within an individual. It helps you make better decisions, improve relationships, and find your purpose.
6. **The Enneagram System:** This system describes nine personality types and their paths to growth. It is designed to understand core motivations, fears, and behaviour patterns, offering a path for personal growth and deeper self-awareness.

7. **Past Life Regression Therapy:** Explore past lives to understand recurring behaviours and emotions.

8. **Shadow Work**: Based on Carl Jung's concept of the 'shadow,' this practice involves examining repressed aspects of oneself. It fosters self-acceptance and growth by integrating the psyche's 'darker' parts. We have a whole chapter on this next.

9. **Contemplation Practices**: Over time, people can reveal profound truths about their core essence by exploring questions like 'Who am I beyond my roles and thoughts?'

10. **Soul Retrieval or Shamanic Healing**: Parts of the soul may be 'lost' due to trauma. These techniques aim to recover those parts, providing a sense of wholeness. I have never experienced shamanic healing, but this makes sense to me in that if there are too many shadows (traumas/emotions) in the body, the soul has less room, and to truly heal of these would add space for your soul and light to shine. This space would allow us to be who our soul wants us to be. Be careful if you go down this path, as not all healers are in the light.

11. **Body-mind practices** (e.g., yoga, tai chi, and qigong): Connecting with the body through these practices can surface hidden feelings, memories, or truths, offering insights into more profound self-awareness.

12. **Ikigai:** This Japanese philosophy encourages individuals to find their 'reason for being' by combining what they love, what they're good at, what the world needs, and what they can be rewarded for. Thus, it fosters purpose and alignment with one's values. While researching this book, I encountered

several Japanese philosophies and customs, and I have to say they know what they're doing.

13. **Journaling and Automatic Writing are ways** to connect with the inner self. These practices allow spontaneous thoughts and feelings to emerge, revealing one's inner identity layers.

14. **Dream Analysis**: By exploring recurring symbols and themes in dreams, people can uncover parts of their subconscious that inform the conscious self.

Each method helps you discover more about yourself and your deepest motivations. Some are looking at you on a deep level. Others are just looking at your personality and quirks. Who you are today could be very different from who you are next year, so take the personality ones with a grain of salt. Of course, there are countless more options out there, but these are the ones I'm most familiar with. What made you think, 'Ooh, I'd love to try that'? Follow that little spark; it's probably lighting the path you're meant to take. I'm not saying you should dive into all these tools like it's an all-you-can-eat buffet. Just pick one or two that resonate with you or none at all! You can get to know yourself without them; sometimes, quiet times in nature can reveal the most amazing insights.

The Many Aspects of You

There are so many parts to who we are; we possess multiple aspects. Think of all the aspects of you: work you, partner you, parent you, friend you, sibling you, party person you, child you, and the list goes on. Understanding yourself reflects the process of knowing many parts. We have different aspects of ourselves that come out in various situations. Consider the different parts of who you are, recognising the many selves that coexist within you. Reflect on how you shift depending on whom you're with.

This example might resonate with you, or you might know someone similar. Nathan is a total perfectionist at work, and because of this, he became a bit of a workaholic. He is constantly striving for flawless outcomes and pushing himself to exceed expectations. Nathan knows he takes things too far, and his co-workers don't enjoy him. Nathan is exhausted, but he can't help it. He has always said that it's just the way he is. After reading a post on social media one day, something triggered Nathan, and he started on a journey of self-exploration. He began by taking the time to analyse parts of himself, the most prominent part being his work self. 'Work Nathan,' he realised, was detrimental to his health and lifestyle, just like the practice of contemplation from the list of self-exploration tools we described above. He became a detective of himself, writing a multitude of questions. What belief am I holding about myself or the world? Where might this belief come from? What do I fear would happen if I make a mistake or fail at something at work? When did I first feel the need to be perfect? What was happening in my life at that time? What would it mean about me if I didn't meet my high standards? Am I motivated by a desire for excellence or a fear of failure? What am I sacrificing in my life to maintain this perfectionism? How do I want my work colleagues to see me? What activates happiness or unworthiness in me at work? He just kept asking questions until he got to the core. He eventually discovered that his perfectionism was from a deep-seated fear of rejection or failure. How did it get there? He traced it to childhood; he only received attention or validation when he achieved top grades or excelled in activities. Over time, his self-worth became tied to external achievements. He now carries an inner belief that creates inadequacy or unworthiness, probably because of being criticised or punished for errors in the past. Now, as an adult, his fears manifest as perfectionism. He believes it protects him from negative outcomes like disappointment, judgment, or even job loss. This perfectionism is actually how he has been protecting himself. It functions as a type of shield to protect him from external threats. Although this drive has led to professional success, it has also come at a cost: stress, burnout and inability to delegate. Knowing this part of himself, he began working on the steps in the upcoming chapters of this book. This work created space for his personal life, lessening his self-inflicted pressure. Nathan changed his life path with the work he put in. Where is he now? He is still very successful, his work colleagues can see a much lighter him, and he has saved himself some future health problems. Additionally, he's found time for romance and a significant other. Don't we love a happy ending?

If you have some revelations about yourself, don't fret; we will delve into the remedy steps in later chapters. This chapter is all about getting to know yourself and the many fascinating (and occasionally frustrating) parts of you. Here's the thing: if you can't pinpoint the root cause of a trait that's throwing your life out of balance, it's not a big deal. Uncovering the 'why' doesn't always require a full excavation. What's important is that you're becoming more self-aware. As these patterns come into focus, you'll find they begin to balance themselves out, like shining a flashlight in a dark room and realising the monster is just a coat rack. It's about recognising the different versions of yourself in various situations and understanding how they shape your experience.

We often show different sides of ourselves depending on who we're with or our situation. These varied selves come with their own unique emotional landscapes. Do you find you have certain emotions coming up with particular people? A person may trigger you and activate an emotion that has been lying dormant for years that you had no idea about. Usually, these triggers appear in romantic relationships but may also pop up in a job or anywhere. It is because you are being exposed to something that activates a memory, a memory you may have suppressed and hidden behind a protective shield in your subconscious. We will delve into releasing hidden emotions later in the book. Until we get there, pay attention and reflect on when these emotions may come up, and write them down. Think of these times as blessings; you needed these emotions to come up so you could heal them.

Remember to honour all parts of yourself, even the messy or destructive ones. Many frustrating traits stem from protective emotions and beliefs. Remember the inner protective shield Nathan was holding? The self-protective shield may be essential for you for a period. And let's not forget the positive aspects of you because, believe me, not everything is a fix-it project! Take the time to identify and value your unique strengths; they are key to your growth and well-being and inspire others.

Know Thyself

A Bit of Ancient History

Why should we get to know all these parts of us? The term *'Know Thyself'* originates from Ancient Greece, inscribed at the Temple of Apollo at Delphi around the 6th Century BC. This simple yet profound phrase reminded visitors that understanding oneself was essential before seeking knowledge or guidance from the divine (the Field). Back then, they were onto something. Self-awareness wasn't just encouraged; it was considered sacred. Instead of looking inward, we are programmed to focus on the external. Nowadays, it's more about chasing likes, achievements and other people's opinions. However, self-discovery elim*i*nates the need for external approval; we ignore irrelevant opinions in *Opposite World*. We stop chasing the feeling of incompleteness because we realise, wait for it … you've been whole all along. Let's be honest: Who stands by you through every moment, from triumphs to trials, laughter to tears? The person I am referring to is none other than you. Always you.

A Greek philosopher, Socrates, was famous for saying, 'The unexamined life is not worth living.' He believed true wisdom came from recognising ignorance and constantly questioning our beliefs, values and actions. Using his famous questioning method, Socrates guided people to self-understanding. But his commitment to self-awareness and truth wasn't popular with everyone. The powers of the time found his ideas threatening, accusing him of corrupting the youth and disrespecting the gods. His radical thinking resulted in a death sentence. How brutal is that? I guess if he lived in our time, he would have been censored on social media, or he would have been considered crazy rather than killed.

The story of Socrates reminds us that learning about ourselves is a journey that changes us but can also be challenging. There will always be those who judge people for thinking outside the box, but that's a sign you're on the right path. In *Opposite World*, we're the minority, and that's totally OK; who wants to be the same as everyone else? I know I don't.

As morbid as it is, history is filled with individuals who tried to guide others toward self-awareness and enlightenment, only to face repression, censorship or persecution. They knew back then that knowing yourself was the only path to wholeness. I commend those brave individuals working to empower the public through self-awareness, and I will list just a few of them below.

- **Jesus of Nazareth (Yeshua) (c. 4 BC–30/33 AD)** Taught that *'The kingdom of God is within you'* (Luke 17:21), emphasising self-awareness and our connection to the divine without the need for intermediaries. While religious institutions later built hierarchical systems, Yeshua taught direct access to the Divine (the Field). His teachings encouraged people to cultivate their connection through faith, love, and self-awareness—rather than relying on religious authorities. His revolutionary teachings challenged religious authorities and societal norms, resulting in his crucifixion.

- **Hypatia of Alexandria (c. 360–415 AD)** This teacher and philosopher examined the world and ourselves through self-reflection and critical thinking. Her teachings threatened religious powers, and a mob murdered her.

- **Giordano Bruno (1548–1600)** A philosopher who believed in an infinite universe and the divinity within all beings, aligning with self-discovery. His radical ideas led to his execution by burning at the stake.

- **Galileo Galilei (1564–1642)** Beyond his science, Galileo showed how questioning what we believe helps us know ourselves better. His advocacy for evidence-based truth led to house arrest by the Church.

- **Carl Jung (1875–1961)** Focused on the *shadow self* and self-awareness, encouraging people to explore their unconscious mind. Although he was not persecuted (phew), critics often dismissed his ideas as too spiritual for mainstream psychology.

- **Dr. Wilhelm Reich (1897–1957)** Explored emotional and energetic health as a pathway to self-awareness and challenging societal norms. Reich's controversial ideas led to the banning of his books, and he ultimately died in prison.

These fantastic teachers all lived in *Opposite Worlds* in their time. Their desire to empower others through truth, critical thinking, and self-knowledge was the thread connecting them, often challenging societal norms or institutions. If they lived in our time instead of being burned at the stake, crucified, or exiled, they would face a modern 'cancel culture' or viral backlash on social media. They would also probably be called conspiracy theorists. Before you call someone that, do you know where the term came from? The term originated in the 1960s and was associated with the CIA, which allegedly used it in internal communications to discredit critics and sceptics of the official explanation of the JFK assassination, framing them as untrustworthy or irrational. Most of us living in *Opposite World* might be labelled conspiracy theorists because we dare to think beyond the programming of the masses.

So, let's honour the courage of these great teachers by ensuring their efforts weren't in vain. Their sacrifices were for a timeless truth: the importance of self-awareness. Don't beat yourself up if you haven't gotten to know yourself. Our schooling and upbringing focus on teaching us about the external world. Now you know it's time to discover your true self, and you will find the key to unlock your boundless *possibilities*.

I want to draw your attention to a caveat that applies to all the chapters in this book: the distinction between knowledge and wisdom and the gap between knowing something and embodying it. I explained this concept in the introduction, but it's essential, so I'll mention it again. Knowledge is the understanding and accumulation of facts, concepts and tools. Wisdom means integrating knowledge with one's authentic self. This book's information is useless unless you align the knowledge with your life. Too many people walk around wearing masks and saying all the right things but not living by them. In *Opposite World*, we are in sync with our true selves.

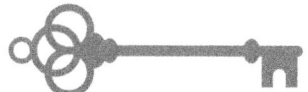

To change your world, know yourself.

My Highest Values

We're about to dive into an exercise to help you uncover your highest values. *Why bother?* Well, for a lot of good reasons, but here's the big one: when it comes to manifesting, if what you're trying to call in from the Field doesn't align with your core values, it's like trying to tune into your favourite song on the wrong radio frequency — it just won't click, it's a 'no match'! Another big reason is that everything you do must align with your values if you want to feel authentic and fulfilled — think about jobs, friendships, studies, and the choices you make every day. How can you do that, though, if you don't even know what your highest values are? What exactly does 'highest values' mean? Your highest values are the things that matter most to you, the core principles or priorities that guide your decisions and make you feel fulfilled. Knowing your values is like having a compass that aligns you with what truly resonates with you. So, let's figure out what lights you up and sets your soul's GPS to *'Yes, please.'* In *Opposite World*, we stay true to our values in every area of life, even if it means our circles shrink, and we must say 'no' more often.

In today's world, people often let outside influences dictate what they value. Here's the truth: Absolute alignment comes from knowing what matters most to you. Let's take a few moments to discover your core values. It's simpler than you think and might change how you see yourself. You may have already come up with it while reading earlier parts of this chapter.

STEP 1: BRAINSTORM YOUR VALUES

Here is a list of common values to get you started. Choose ten and let intuition guide you. If a value you love isn't on the list, feel free to add it!

Curiosity	Kindness	Love
Service	Trust	Wellness
Responsibility	Humour	Freedom
Security	Bravery	Wealth
Purpose	Achievement	Happiness
Peace	Family	Faith
Playfulness	Adventure	Fairness
Balance	Fame	Growth
Harmony	Justice	Learning
Loyalty	Status	Religion
Helping	Stability	Love
Punctuality	Health	Honesty
Creativity	Tidiness	Fun
Sympathy	Reliability	Quality
Hard Work	Decisiveness	Protection

STEP 2: PICK YOUR TOP 5

From the ten words you picked, narrow them down to five (5) words.

Hint: Ask yourself: *Which of these values feel essential to who I am?*

STEP 3: RANK YOUR TOP 5

Now, rank your top 5 in order of importance. Your #1 value will likely be the foundation of everything you stand for.

STEP 4: REFLECT ON YOUR VALUE/S

Take a moment to think about your values. Ask yourself:

- *How have my values shaped my decisions, relationships, or goals?*
- *When have I felt most in alignment with my values?*
- *When have I felt frustrated or stuck — was it because my values weren't being honoured?*
- *What could I change to live in alignment with my values?*

Understanding your values isn't just about self-discovery; it's about creating a life that aligns with who you are at your core.

When your values align with your choices, life feels smoother, like you're swimming with the current instead of against it.

And remember, your values are your compass. If you don't take the time to set your direction, someone else will happily do it for you. So, take charge, and start living a life that's true to you.

I haven't reinvented the wheel here; plenty of people teach how to discover one's core values. If you haven't landed on a clear answer yet, don't stress! Keep exploring. You might find some online tools that can help.

Once you've found your main value word (or words), please write it down. Pin it somewhere you'll see it often. And most importantly, live your life in a way that embodies it. After all, your values aren't just something to *know* but something to *be*. If you are going for a job or hanging out with friends, stop and consider if you are aligning with your highest value. This awareness may give you some key advice.

The Life Alignment Tracker

We have examined our internal selves. Now, let us examine our external lives. It helps to assess how balanced your life feels. Imagine your life as a wheel with different sections; if some areas thrive while others are flat, the ride gets bumpy. Below is a quick check-in to see where things might feel shaky.

Take a moment to rate how satisfied you feel in each area of your life on a scale of 1 to 10, where one means 'needs a lot of love' and ten means 'nailed it!' Remember, this is a personal exercise, so your rating should reflect how you feel inside, not what others might think. For example, if you're not in a romantic relationship, that doesn't automatically mean you should give it a zero; you might be perfectly content flying solo right now, and singleton is probably precisely where you should be. Or you may not have a billion dollars, but you are happy and comfortable and have no desire for more money. It's about where you are and what feels right for you. We are all on our unique paths.

Relationship (Romantic)	
Social Life	
Fun	
Finance	
Physical Health	
Family	
Boundaries	
Alone Time	
Career	
Emotional Health	
Personal Growth & Spirituality	

Spotting the Bumpy Areas

Once you've put a number against each area, take a step back. Which areas feel solid? Which needs attention? The idea isn't to aim for perfection; it's about creating a life that feels balanced for you. For instance, you might thrive in your career and finances but struggle with your health or emotions. Think of workaholic Nathan; when he did this exercise, most of his areas were assessed as low, besides his career, well, at least until he worked on that. He did this exercise again six months later, and it was a much more balanced wheel. Recognising those gaps allows you to bring more balance into your life. Even one slight shift in a low-scoring area can change your overall harmony. This exercise is a powerful way to reflect on the big picture of your life. It might reveal significant areas for improvement or even inspire deep gratitude for accomplishments you should be proud of.

If you like, you can transfer these numbers to a visual circle, like the one below. Shade it in, write the numbers, or use it in whatever way works for you. This simple visual can help you see where your life feels balanced and where there's room for growth.

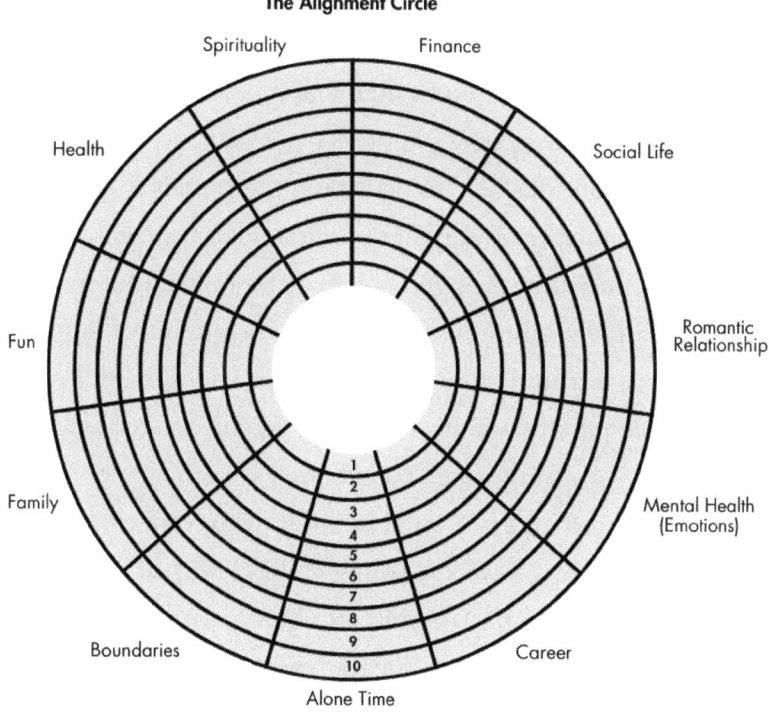

By spotting the gaps, you can uncover where your life feels out of sync. No guilt trips, just a gentle nudge toward creating a life that genuinely reflects who you are.

Feel free to skip to the next chapter if you feel well-balanced in all areas and genuinely can't see room for improvement after this little activity. But if you've spotted areas that could use a little more love, let's take a moment to explore some of the common aspects of life that people struggle with. Areas like health, spirituality and emotions will be covered in later chapters. For now, we will look at finance and relationships, the two areas most people focus on. Who knows? Something might trigger a lightbulb moment for you.

Reflection - 'What's one small thing I can do this week to feel more aligned in the least balanced area?'

Money Mindset

In the early 2000s, I taught financial investment courses. What stood out was that people's mindsets, not bank accounts, were the most significant obstacle to achieving their goals. I quickly realised that no matter how great their financial strategies were, they would fail until they changed how they thought about money. So, I started adding mindset sections to the beginning of my courses long before this kind of education became widespread. I returned to the basics of why we think, feel, speak, and act in specific ways. It's mostly programming. Your belief system sits in your subconscious mind and is shaped by those who 'programmed' you, especially when you were a young child. Think of your subconscious like a computer running on old software — that's loaded with apps and files over the years, and some of them start running randomly in the background. The problem (or perhaps it's a blessing) is that it doesn't know fact from fiction; it just repeats what it has learned. The good news? We can uninstall some of this outdated programming and rewrite it. It takes time because those old files have been there for so long, but self-awareness is the first step. In the following chapters, we'll dive into how to rewire programming that doesn't do us any favours.

Do you have negative programming around money? A quick way to uncover limiting beliefs is by looking within:

Finish these sentences:

'People with money are _____.'

'I would have more money if _____.'

'My parents thought money was _____.'

'Money causes _____.'

Let's face it: If you don't like rich people, how will you attract money?

I call negative money programming the 'scarcity mindset.' I used to call it 'poor man syndrome,' but I think that was a bit rude. If these sayings feel uncomfortable, take a moment to reflect. This book is about being brave enough to face yourself. This term describes a pattern of focusing on negatives, such as saying, 'I can't afford it,' or 'Money doesn't grow on trees,' or experiencing feelings of jealousy when others succeed. These beliefs can trap us in a cycle of lack and reinforce a sense of victimhood. Awareness is the first step to breaking free and opening yourself up to abundance. While not everyone starts from the same place, shifting our mindset can help us create new opportunities and possibilities within our circumstances. We cannot tune in to the abundance frequency if we have blocks holding us back.

Here's the truth: thinking about money isn't greedy. In *Opposite World*, we flip the way we think about money. It's not something to fear, hate, or avoid — it's simply energy in motion. Like all energy, it flows where it's directed. When used with intention, money can be deeply spiritual. It creates opportunities, supports loved ones, and, when directed consciously, becomes a force for positive change. Wanting more isn't selfish; it's about expanding your capacity to give, grow, and live fully.

We need to be on the same frequency as abundance to attract it. If this challenges you, take the time to work on shifting these beliefs before manifesting or meditating money into your life. Start with straightforward changes. For example, if you catch yourself saying, 'I can't afford that,' shift it to 'How can I afford that?'. Or when you are paying your electricity bill, instead of feeling stressed, think how grateful you are for the light and power. In *the Opposite World*, we think and believe in the opposite. As we have already discussed, everything is energy, and money is energy. The more you resist money, think negatively about it, or see it as something you'll never have enough of, the more you reinforce that reality. Energy flows where attention goes; if your energy around money is full of frustration or fear, those feelings will be reflected back to you. Just as we explained in the Field, this rule applies to everything. So, focus on shifting your energy toward appreciating money, even in small ways. Start by noticing how money supports you daily, whether it's the coffee you enjoyed this morning, your clothes, or the roof over your head. When you change your energy from resistance to gratitude, you'll be amazed at how things start to shift. Unexpected opportunities, gifts, and solutions may appear out of nowhere. It's not magic; it's alignment. When you feel good about money, you naturally attract more, and life seems to work out in your favour. We will learn how to generate abundance in this book, so nail this mindset step if necessary.

Romantic Relationships

Relationships are a massive topic! Honestly, I could write an entire book on this alone. Romantic relationships have this uncanny way of shining a spotlight on our shadows, bringing all those hidden parts of ourselves to the surface. But here's the thing: they can also be one of your life's most incredible growth opportunities if you're willing to face and own those reflections instead of pointing fingers. Relationships are like holding up a mirror: scary, enlightening, and sometimes hilarious, all at once. On the contrary, if you are in a healthy relationship that matches your values, parts of you will come out and shine.

Whether you're hoping to be in one or want to improve the one you're in, relationships are an area most people focus on. Suppose you've rated this part of your life low, maybe because you're single or your current relationship feels more like a reality TV show than a love story. Either way, it's important to remember that your romantic life isn't the sole ingredient in a meaningful life. We are better off not being in one than being in one that destroys our soul.

For younger readers, you probably don't need to dive too deep into this; read on and stick this wisdom in your back pocket for later.

As we've discussed, relationships can act as mirrors for our shadows, pulling us toward people who reflect our fears or align with our current frequency. If this is an area you're struggling with, it might be time to turn that mirror inward and ask, 'What is this trying to teach me?'

Here's a truth pill to swallow: expecting a partner to fill the holes in your happiness is a fast track to disappointment. No one can make you feel a certain way — that's your job. Healthy relationships flourish when two people come together as whole beings, not two halves trying to complete a jigsaw.

Speaking of jigsaws, have you seen the stand-up show *Jigsaw* by Daniel Sloss? It's hilarious but also scarily accurate. Sloss describes his show as not being anti-relationships but that he hates 90% of them. In his brutally honest style, he talks about how people pretend to be happy and settle for mediocrity in relationships. With 9 billion people on the planet, why stay in a relationship that doesn't fulfil you? The impact of *Jigsaw* has been profound. Since its release in 2018, it is said that over 250,000 breakups, 300 divorces, and countless cancelled engagements have been attributed to it. Sloss challenges societal pressures to stay in unsatisfying relationships and invites viewers to rethink what they truly want. You can find *Jigsaw* streaming on Netflix if you're ready for a laugh and maybe a life-changing perspective. Remember, until you face the parts of your life that are out of alignment, you won't be a frequency match with *Opposite World*.

If, in your heart, you know you're somewhere your soul doesn't belong, it's time to pause and ask yourself the hard questions.

What are you holding onto?
What are you afraid to let go of?
Are you putting all your pain onto your partner, expecting them to fix what's broken inside you?
Are the dynamics not working?
Are you struggling to breathe in the relationship?
Have you lost your true self?

Did you have any lightbulb moments while reading these questions? Is it time to find a path that allows both of you the time to grow and heal? If you drop into *Opposite World*, where thinking differently creates real change, a rekindling of love might blossom

... or maybe not. Either way, you'll find clarity and alignment with your soul's needs.

Are you getting over a breakup and going through the 'I've wasted time being with this person' phase? Stop. It was a blessing. Allow yourself to see this blessing; you have been given an opportunity to learn something about yourself. We are often drawn to people for a reason, and sometimes, it's to shine a light on our hidden emotions. Whether it is to uncover hidden emotions (stay tuned to next chapter), guide you on a different path, or show you what you want, it's always a blessing.

Before you work on your current relationship or dream about a future partner, the number one relationship you need to nurture is the one with yourself. Loving yourself at a soul level isn't about chanting affirmations in the mirror like 'I love me' (although, no harm if you want to). It's about cultivating a deep, unshakable feeling of love for who you are. And that takes time.

When you genuinely love yourself, you become your own best company. Take yourself out on dates, treat yourself with kindness, and embody the qualities you hope to find in a partner. The irony is that the more whole and fulfilled you feel, the more likely you are to attract a relationship that reflects that same depth and love.

And if you're already in a relationship? Learning to love yourself can shift everything. As your frequency changes, it naturally influences the people in your field. Your partner might pick up on that higher vibration and evolve alongside you.

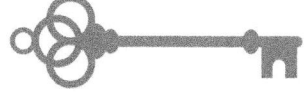

Wholeness starts within – love yourself first, and the rest will fall into place.

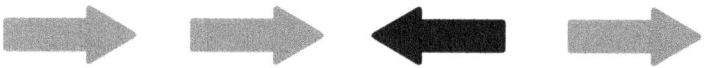

CHAPTER 4

UNMASKING THE SILENT SHADOWS WITHIN

STEP 2

What is preventing you from achieving your dreams?

Letting the Light In

In step 1, we explored who we are, what makes us shine and what dims our light. You may have uncovered some emotions that fuel negative behaviours or energies in your life. Did anything uncomfortable pop up for you? Was there a flicker of unease when we delved into the mirrors within ourselves or when we touched on money and relationships? Your hidden shadows may just be waving hello, ready for you to notice them. In this chapter, we will delve deeper into these emotions and discover how to let them go. I'll be honest; this is a heavy but essential topic, so we'll work through it as lightly as possible. A key thing many people overlook when they meditate or manifest is the potential blocks obstructing their path. On the flip side to negative emotions or traits, did you get to know some great qualities about yourself that you previously failed to appreciate? I hope so; if not, look harder because there are many. The more you love parts of yourself, the more the other parts shine.

Here's the thing: you don't need to over-analyse where these emotional blocks come from. Some people spend far too much time untangling their dark shadows, trying to piece together every thread of their past. For some, the source of their pain might be obvious — big traumas often are. But for others, it could be a vague sense of fear, inadequacy or unworthiness with no clear origin. And guess what? It doesn't always matter. This block could stem from a past life or ancestral burden. Shadows can sometimes appear with no standout reason. For instance, your underlying unworthiness could stem from something so minor. Like when Johnny, in first grade, laughed at you because you couldn't tie your shoelace, or Helen, in grade two, who bullied you for picking your nose … but it was just a scratch. Could it be possible that being rejected by Jeremy in 5th grade is causing you to seek validation through social media likes or staying in unhealthy relationships? Of course, I'm oversimplifying here and using basic examples, for only you know you. In *Opposite World*, where transformation is the goal, we don't cling to those shadows; we release them.

Why should we face our trapped emotions or silent shadows? Why don't we leave them alone? Because these blocks usually don't just sit silently in the background, they can wreak havoc on your mental, emotional, and even physical health. They can be silent little suckers for years and then spring out in some form at various stages of your life. Left unchecked, they may manifest as stress, anxiety, chronic pain, or even illness. And here's the sneaky part: we can become addicted to them. Our body is wired to what's familiar; it clings to these blocks like an old security blanket, even when they cause us harm.

Okay, you acknowledge that some work might be necessary, but how do you set them free? How do we clear this bridge that offers freedom and access to the Field? We will work through some tools to feel them and then set them free. Letting go of blocks (emotions) can feel impossible when they've been with you for so long because, to you, they feel normal. Perhaps these lower emotions have been a familiar aspect of your emotional state for a while. That's why, in this chapter, we'll explore simple tools to help you dissolve them. The last thing you want is to stay stuck, clinging to the weight of a story that no longer serves you. You've already done the first step, and that is to acknowledge them. Awareness is everything.

It won't always be easy and is going to take some courage. At times, this journey may feel uncomfortable, even confronting. Why? Because your body will resist, it wants to stay how it is, even to your detriment. On the contrary, it's one of the most rewarding and life-changing things you will ever do. And on the other side? Freedom, clarity, and a version of yourself that feels whole and unshakable. You will feel lighter than ever, and joy and love will pour out of you. The lightness you will hold will allow space for any new creations you wish for.

What Are Emotions?

An emotion is an energy-driven response that reflects how we perceive and react to experiences, connecting our thoughts, bodies, and feelings. Our subconscious operates like a computer running outdated programs. Emotions are tied to these programs. These emotions can be low-frequency emotions like unworthiness, self-doubt, and fear. Emotions can be automatic and unconscious, meaning you might not even realise they're there. Just like our body is energy, as we explored in the chapter The Field, so too are emotions. They carry vibrations that can align us with higher states or keep us stuck in patterns. Remember Nathan in the earlier chapter? Nathan had some outdated programs that appeared different in his outer world. Once he went down and met his underlying trapped emotions and did the work, many things changed in his world because his surrounding energy changed. Releasing his fear of not measuring up improved the balance and realism of his work life. He met a wonderful partner and became closer to his family. He had not focused on fixing any of these parts of his life, but they came together by changing his frequency. Nathan is now happily engaged to Trish, who shares his love for this inner work. He would never have met her without releasing his suppressed emotions because he would not have matched her frequency. Even if you focus on improving one aspect of your life, unexpected bonuses may pop up in other areas.

Like Nathan's story, let me share a personal story on how working on your inner self can change areas you didn't expect. For years, I worked diligently on clearing internal emotions and felt confident that I had released most of the negative ones. Then, something unexpected happened during a retreat where I meditated for hours daily. By day seven, I observed that a slight yet constant anxiety, so subtle that I hadn't ever acknowledged its presence, had disappeared. It had lingered in the background for so long, shaping my inner world without ever surfacing fully. It was like a shadow in stealth mode, lurking just out of sight, waiting in the woods. And then, as if by magic, it was simply ... gone. A few days after the retreat, I experienced another profound shift. Standing on the edge of a high cliff overlooking the ocean, I realised my fear of heights had disappeared. My toes weren't tingling, and instead of the usual hesitation, I leaned over to take in the view. It was an extreme change for me and completely unintentional. I hadn't been working on this fear; it wasn't even on my radar. So, what happened? This quiet shadow, this hidden fragment of emotion, had been released. Not because I focused on it but because I spent hours each day immersed in love, heart coherence, and connecting with the Field.

As you can see from my examples, a bonus to making any changes in your life is that some unexpected things may happen that you didn't expect. Keep this in mind as we continue through the chapters. Hopefully, you understand why we are focusing on these steps. These hidden shadows affect our outlook on life, personality and the frequencies we emit into the world. They can also dramatically impact our health.

The Connection Between Emotions and Health

The fascinating thing about emotions is that they don't just live in your mind but also your body. Scientists have found that emotions like anger and sadness can imprint physically on the body. These imprints influence body systems like your heart rate, hormones, and immune system. Emotions aren't just 'feelings'; they're energy in motion, meant to flow through and out of us. The problem arises when we hold on to them, allowing blocks to form, which can manifest as physical or emotional distress. One striking example of this mind-body connection is the phenomenon known as 'broken heart syndrome.' When someone experiences profound emotional grief, such as losing a loved one, their heart can suffer physical damage. Heartbreak isn't just metaphorical; it's an actual condition called takotsubo cardiomyopathy, where the heart muscle temporarily weakens under the weight of stress hormones. Studies show a link between severe grief and a higher risk of heart problems. These studies demonstrate that unprocessed emotions don't merely linger; they significantly affect our physical health, highlighting the importance of emotional release.

Our bodies are extraordinarily intelligent and capable of so much more than we often give them credit for. Remember, in Chapter 1, we explored how our bodies consist primarily of energy. So, doesn't it make sense to consider working on health issues from an energetic level rather than focusing on the dense, 3D world of matter? I want to rephrase that: if our bodies are mainly energy, doesn't it make sense to approach healing from an energetic perspective, not just the physical?

I mentioned earlier in the chapter that many people suffer from health anxiety. What is that? It's when you constantly fear you have a health issue. Unfortunately, being in that frequency mirrors it back to you. Think of it like this: what you fear, you create. Much of our health anxiety stems from a system that often operates on fear. I am not rejecting Western medicine; it excels in emergencies and acute situations. There is, however, a broader perspective on how we view and care for our bodies. It's also about giving you your power so you don't feel this fear. Growth requires us to think outside the box, to challenge the familiar, and to explore unconventional ideas.

Take a moment to reflect on these three upcoming concepts I will put forward. Step outside of your usual programming and view them with fresh eyes. These concepts might be entirely new to you, and I am not writing them to be controversial. Instead, I hope they will empower you, especially if you're facing illness or grappling with health anxiety.

1. **Contagious Diseases** — Research shows that almost 80% of diseases are non-communicable, meaning they cannot be spread from person to person. So, most people are not suffering from something they have caught from someone else but instead have a chronic illness with the leading causes being stress (including trapped emotions), environmental toxins, and lifestyle choices. These diseases contribute to the majority of deaths, and because they are not contagious, we have a great deal of preventative control over them. This information empowers us to question much of what we've been taught about illness and recognise our influence over our health. But what about the remaining 20-26% of diseases that are communicable? Should we hide in a bunker to avoid being in the 20% category? Even these contagious diseases

can be prevented or minimised by boosting overall health and immunity. A healthy body is better able to fight off or prevent illness.

I believe that the core of most illnesses is our internal emotional state, which is why this chapter is so important. And guess what? Disease and ill health thrive on low-vibe emotions like fear.

2. **Germ Theory vs. Terrain Theory** — Louis Pasteur first explained the germ theory of disease in the 1860s. Claude Bernard and Antoine Béchamp introduced the terrain theory in the late 19th century. Let's look at these two theories. The germ theory states that microorganisms cause illness by invading our bodies. The terrain theory suggests that a healthy and balanced internal environment makes the body resistant to infection. In other words, you can't 'catch' anything if your mind and body are in harmony. But here's the twist: It is rumoured that Pasteur admitted this on his deathbed: 'The microbe is nothing; the terrain is everything.' This confession aligns him with the terrain theory, even though he discovered the germ theory.

Wouldn't it make more sense to focus on preventative health instead of waiting for symptoms to appear? Wouldn't it be better to keep your terrain as clean as possible by eliminating toxins (poisons) and keeping your body as stress-free as possible?

3. **Most Diseases Are Not Inherited** — What about diseases you've been told are genetic? Are you doomed if you have a disease in the family? Not at all. I want to introduce

you to epigenetics. It shows that most diseases once thought to be purely genetic are not. The word epigenetics comes from the Greek prefix 'epi', which means above or on top of. So, epigenetics literally means 'above genetics'. Epigenetics shows that only a handful of diseases are strictly inherited. Examples include Huntington's disease, cystic fibrosis and sickle cell anaemia. Specific genetic mutations cause the diseases listed. As discussed above, most common diseases, like heart disease, diabetes, and cancer, are largely influenced by lifestyle, stress, toxins, and nutrition. Epigenetics shows us that environmental factors can turn on or turn off specific genes.

Epigenetics explains that your genes are not your destiny; you have control over how they are expressed through your thoughts, choices and environment. Understanding epigenetics can help with your belief that you can heal your body on a cellular level. I recommend Bruce Lipton's work if you want to dive deep into epigenetics. In my eyes, he's the king of this field.

Hopefully, those three health concepts will help you view your body differently. It's not just your physical body but also your emotional state that keeps you healthy. As discussed in the chapter about heart coherence, stress hormones like cortisol and adrenaline are designed to help us in short-term emergencies; this is no problem for the body. The real issue is that stress hormones are constantly flooding our bodies. Modern life pressures and unresolved and trapped emotions fuel this cycle. The more stress hormones we produce, the more our bodies adapt to them, ultimately losing the ability to heal. This vicious cycle continues until we become addicted to the very hormones that are damaging us.

It's like being stuck on a never-ending treadmill. These trapped emotions can manifest into countless symptoms and diseases. Wouldn't it make sense to cultivate a calm inner world to prevent or even heal these health issues? Guess what? You have the power to stop this cycle.

What if we stepped into *Opposite World* and became the commander of our own body? By acknowledging and releasing these emotional blocks, we could break free from our cycles, calm our stress response, and heal emotionally, which can also heal us physically. Why not give it a go? It's not going to harm you. Let's try to address trapped emotions before seeking medication to suppress them because they come with possible side effects (like anxiety and depression … go figure). To be clear, there are absolutely situations where medications are essential, especially for those experiencing acute or severe conditions. However, it's important to remember that these medications don't address the root cause of the problem. They may be essential to manage life temporarily, but the underlying issue remains. If we continually mask our emotions, how can we ever feel them deeply enough to release them? **We need to feel to heal!** By exploring these layers of healing, we open the door to more lasting and meaningful change.

Opening your eyes to this information is the first step towards reclaiming or controlling your health. In *Opposite World*, we step into our power as the true masters of our bodies. Remember, your thoughts and emotions are mirrors. So, next time you hear yourself say, '*Bad knees just run in the family, so I'm bound to get them,*' remember your body is listening to that. You have more power than you give yourself credit for. In my next chapter, I will tell you a story of how I created symptoms just from thoughts alone.

~

Have you heard of German new medicine (GNM)? One of the most fascinating medical doctors I've encountered is Dr Ryke Geerd Hamer, a German practitioner and the founder of GNM. His work explores the profound connection between emotional shocks and physical health. Dr. Hamer's research began after he developed testicular cancer following the traumatic loss of his son, Dirk, who was shot in 1978. This personal experience prompted Dr. Hamer to explore the relationship between emotional shocks and disease.

He analysed around 31,000 patients' histories and brain scans during his research. He identified clear correlations between specific emotional conflicts, corresponding regions of the brain, and their related manifestations in the body. I'll explain that in simple terms: he observed that when someone experienced a strong emotional shock or conflict, scans showed a visible mark in specific areas of the brain. These brain areas were directly connected to specific body parts and could show up as physical symptoms or illnesses in those areas. An example relating to his personal experience was his discovery that testicular cancer traced back to 'profound loss' or 'loss conflicts,' such as the death of a child.

To completely flip things to the Opposite, German new medicine also explains that symptoms experienced by the body are signs it has entered the healing phase. The healing phase is when the body is actively repairing and restoring balance following a biological conflict or stress. These findings revolutionise how we view health, showing that it's not something that happens to us but is deeply connected to our internal state. This view differs from Western medicine, which often views symptoms as the onset of an illness rather than a natural part of the body's healing and resolution process.

Dr Hamer's work was heavily criticised by mainstream healthcare, a common experience for those challenging medical norms. I want to point out that humanity can't evolve unless we open our eyes to the limitations within our current knowledge systems. While peer-reviewed studies are often considered the gold standard, it's essential to acknowledge that biases, funding interests, and a reluctance to challenge the status quo influence many of them. History has shown us time and time again that revolutionary ideas are often dismissed, only to transform our understanding of the world many years later. Perhaps it's time we approached such ideas as German new medicine with curiosity and openness rather than outright rejection. Growth often requires the courage to question and explore.

If German new medicine resonates with you, I highly recommend exploring this research. The website is a treasure trove of knowledge and offers incredible insights. Even if you're just curious about an illness or pain you have, you can use the site's directory to explore the potential emotional conflicts behind it. By knowing what conflict matches the area of your body, you can work on clearing the conflict or just being at peace with it. What's the worst that can happen?

So, when it comes to your health, always remember that what feels like a hardware (body) issue might stem from a software (emotion) problem. Our emotions are like hidden codes running in the background, quietly influencing our well-being. They can create patterns of incoherence, stress, tension, and imbalance that directly impact our physical health. By addressing these emotional undercurrents, you may find that the body naturally begins to heal itself. It's a reminder that true wellness is not just about fixing what's broken but also understanding the deeper connections between mind, body, and soul. Emotions aren't obstacles; they're guides, showing you where healing is needed most. So, take time to listen, reflect, and rewrite your inner 'software' to create harmony within. Remember, all diseases resonate at low frequencies. Raise your frequency by following the steps in this book and nurturing heart coherence.

Distractions from Emotions

It's incredible how our emotions can shape our physical health. Unfortunately, many people run from feelings rather than acknowledging them and allowing them to move on. How do people run from them? Distractions. We distract ourselves, avoiding the discomfort of feeling and processing what's going on inside.

Whether through mindless scrolling, binge-watching TV, overeating, working (think Nathan) or staying excessively 'busy' — I'm sure you know someone who is always 'busy', but really, do they need to be? Distractions have become the modern way to escape our inner world, anything to avoid inner pain. Here's the thing about avoiding emotions — it's usually not a conscious decision. Most of us don't wake up thinking, 'Today, I'm going to suppress how I feel.' Instead, the ways we distract ourselves are often subconscious habits. Why do we create distractions? The subconscious mind is wired to avoid pain and seek comfort. These distractions act like a buffer, numbing the discomfort of feeling. In *Opposite World*, we dare to pause, notice these patterns, and ask ourselves, 'What am I really avoiding?'

So many people are terrified of being alone because they don't want to sit with themselves. They do anything to avoid this aloneness by various methods, and a very common one is staying in toxic or unloving relationships. Anything to avoid the discomfort of solitude. But here's the truth: without alone time, you cannot access your true, authentic self.

Take a moment to reflect: Are you distracting yourself from anything? What are you constantly escaping? Here are some other common distractions:

- Alcohol or drugs
- Staying endlessly busy
- Constant drama and chaos
- Wearing a façade or mask (pretending to be someone else)
- Judging or fighting with others (often a reflection of your inner mirror)
- Constantly seeking approval
- Staying in relationships out of fear rather than love
- Overeating or comfort eating
- Being glued to your devices
- Binge-watching TV or endlessly scrolling social media (to escape reality)
- Excessive shopping or spending
- Perfectionism
- Overexercising (pushing the body to avoid mental discomfort)
- Overworking (using work to distract from emotional pain)
- Video gaming or escapism through fantasy worlds
- Overcommitting to others (focusing on everyone else's needs to avoid their own)

- Constantly seeking validation through appearance or achievements
- Clinging to toxic friendships
- Constantly dating new people before ending the last relationship (avoiding time to heal or reflect).

I feel so exhausted just writing that list. Many other distractions exist that I'm sure you could think of.

How often do you hear someone say, I'm giving up alcohol, sugar or whatever? They succeed and feel amazing for a period of time. The next time you see them, they are back to old habits. You wonder, 'How could they go back after how amazing they seemed?'. Why do distractions lure people back? They haven't treated the core problem, so they keep running away — hiding. Think about when you did the alignment life tracker; was there an area you excelled in and others that were not? Perhaps you spend most of your time exercising, but other areas in your life are not so great; are you using exercise or some other distraction as a tool to self-protect?

Instead of running, what if you stopped? What if you allowed yourself to sit with your aloneness, face the brokenness, and uncover the shadows you've been hiding from? Don't be too hard on yourself; these distractions are your subconscious shielding you from pain. Think of these distractions as a band-aid holding everything together; if you lose it, the wound opens back up. Say your distraction is overworking, and then you lose your job. You will fall apart because the job shields you from your shadows. You don't have the resilience you see others have because you haven't learnt to face these hidden emotions.

These distractions may feel comforting in the moment, but on a deep level, it's time they left. If you continue to numb your emotions with these distractions, you will never change who you are. Therefore, your external world will never change. The good news is that you can activate your willpower if you are aware of these distractions.

In *Opposite World*, we don't run from shadows; we dare to face them head-on. Why? Because we know that we are powerful, capable, and liberated when we step into our truth. Then, true healing can happen.

Do any of these distractions ring true to you? Be honest; it's just us here. We've already discussed the importance of knowing yourself, so face it with curiosity rather than fear. Ask yourself this: Are you willing to remove the blindfold and see the world differently? To go all in, decide to change, and commit to yourself today? If your wounds run deep and your distractions are major addictions, it's okay to seek help from an expert. Your body, mind, and soul are worth the effort to clear these blocks.

Ask yourself this question: Do you want to keep escaping the brokenness and hiding from the darkness? Or are you ready to do a clear-out and allow space to let the light in? I hope I know the answer. Keep reading; we are going to do this together.

Releasing Emotions – Feel it to Heal it

Letting go of emotions has been explained by some as feeling like an ego death or experiencing the 'dark night of the soul'. Have you heard of that term? It stems from a 16th-century poem by Saint John of the Cross, describing a soul's journey through deep suffering toward enlightenment. Sounds profound, right?

Releasing emotions isn't easy, but it's transformative and doesn't always happen in one dramatic wave. For some, it's a slow, steady process — chipping away at layers over time. Others, especially those holding deep wounds, might experience a sudden, intense release, often after opening the door through forgiveness, self-compassion, or even a spontaneous breakthrough.

Regardless of the path, the key is to allow emotions to surface entirely rather than suppress them. When you come out the other side, you'll see why every moment of surrender was worth it.

Before we dive into the releasing tool, I would like to introduce Dr. David R. Hawkins. Hawkins is a renowned psychiatrist and spiritual teacher who developed a comprehensive framework for understanding human consciousness. In his book *Letting Go*, he outlines practical steps to help individuals release inner shadows and negative emotions. Dr. Hawkins also introduced the map of consciousness, a scale ranging from 1 to 1,000, which measures various emotional and spiritual states. At the lower end of the scale is shame, calibrated at 20, while the highest level is enlightenment, at 1,000. According to his research, approximately 85% of the world's population calibrates below the critical level of 200, which he identifies as the threshold between destructive and constructive influence. How would you like to step into *Opposite World* and become one of the top 15% of the world with a higher calibration than most people on Earth? Dr. Hawkins's work offers profound insights, and each reading or listening session reveals new layers of understanding. Hawkins conducted extensive research into human consciousness levels across various global regions. His studies suggest, much like the concepts we've discussed regarding the Field and the mirror within, that individuals tend to resonate and harmonise with the emotional frequencies of their environment. Hawkins discovered that areas of high consciousness can elevate individual awareness, positively influencing emotional and spiritual well-being. Conversely, regions with lower levels of consciousness can have the opposite effect, pulling down one's state of mind. His findings reveal the powerful impact of our surroundings on our consciousness, highlighting the importance of choosing environments that nurture our growth and well-being. So perhaps pay attention to where you live or who you hang around. Now that you know this information, consider the impact of specific frequencies on you. Take a moment to reflect on your household or other places in your life. If you're working on letting go of those lower emotions and elevating your frequency, your family members will begin to shift as well, whether they realise it or not. It's like being the Wi-Fi router of good vibes; once you upgrade your signal, everyone in range benefits. And if it doesn't work immediately, at least you're the calm one when someone forgets to put the dishes away!

R.E.L.E.A.S.E – A Tool for Letting Go

Now that you better understand your emotional blocks or potential hidden shadows, let's work on letting them go. I've put together an acronym to guide you in moments of emotional intensity. This tool is built around the word *RELEASE* and is designed to create a calming association when you are in a not-so-calm state. You can use it when you are in a heightened emotion that is not serving you or at any time at all.

R – Remove yourself from the immediate situation

E – Eyes closed and go inward

L – Let your breath slow down

E – Embrace and feel the emotion, exaggerate its intensity

A – Allow this feeling to melt away as you observe it

S – Shift your focus to love and focus on your heart chakra

E – End your session by acknowledging what you are grateful for.

Let me show you how to use this tool. Imagine you're in a fight with a loved one, and suddenly, you're overwhelmed with emotion. Boom, pay attention; something has triggered you. By now, thanks to the work in previous chapters, you recognise this trigger as a clear sign of a trapped emotion bubbling to the surface. Even if you don't know exactly where it came from, that's okay; focus on feeling it and letting it go. You don't need to analyse or overthink it; the magic lies in the simple act of feeling it and releasing it.

Important: Remember to feel the emotion. Feeling emotions is vital, as it allows your body to process the emotional charge, like completing a chemical reaction, helping to neutralise its energy and let it go. Feel it and heal it!

The more you practise, the more it becomes a habit, and the easier letting go will become. If you can't step away when the emotion hits, don't stress. Tuck it into your back pocket and try to revisit it when you have a quiet moment alone. It's all about creating space for yourself to process and release rather than letting those emotions continue to weigh you down. When you finally release them, you will feel much lighter, and your inner light will have more room in your body to guide you.

To Cry or Not to Cry

Here's another tool to help you release emotions. Don't panic, guys. I'm here to share some facts! Crying is one of our body's natural ways to release pent-up emotions. It's often misunderstood as a sign of weakness, but let's be honest: sometimes, life requires a full-on, ugly cry. Those tears serve a purpose, whether over a sad movie, a frustrating day or a traumatic event. When we cry, our brain releases stress-relieving chemicals like endorphins and oxytocin. This release helps us process and calm emotions that might otherwise sit like a heavy backpack on our souls. It's like nature's very own emotional detox; no juice cleanse is required. This release clears out emotional buildup and can ease physical tension and stress stored within the body. Think of it as hitting the emotional reset button, allowing us to move forward with more clarity and a little less baggage. So, when tears come, grab a tissue, maybe two, and let them flow. Your future self will thank you for it.

If you're looking for cultural proof that crying isn't just for toddlers and rom-com addicts, let me introduce you to the Japanese practice of *rui-katsu* (literally meaning 'tear-seeking'). Picture this: groups of people gathering to watch tear-jerking films or listen to gut-wrenching stories on purpose. No, they're not masochists. Rui-katsu is rooted in the idea that crying is good for the soul. It's a chance to let it all out in a safe, communal environment, like therapy but with extra tissues. This practice celebrates the therapeutic benefits of tears, proving that sometimes, sharing a good cry can be as bonding as sharing a laugh. So guys, the next time you get caught tearing up during a rom-com, tell those with you, 'I'm not crying; I'm practising rui-katsu — it's a Japanese self-care ritual. Look it up.'

And now, for the science nerds and curious minds, let's take a deeper dive into the magical mechanics of crying. Water researcher Veider Austin states that your tears are more than just salty water; they're medicine. Here's the fascinating part: our faces are designed so that tears follow a specific path, trickling down our cheeks and into our mouths. It's as though nature intended for us quite literally to taste our emotions. As wild as it sounds, this might be a way for the body to reconnect with the frequency or energy released in those tears, turning them into internal medicine. Austin's research suggests that tears carry emotional frequencies, and releasing them is like purging old, stagnant energy to make room for something lighter.

∼

So, if tears can hold our emotions, what else might act as a vessel for stored feelings? In all its forms, water is more than just a physical substance—it's a carrier of energy and emotion. In the foreword, Dr. Andrew mentioned that it's not just our brain that processes and holds emotions. That idea might be complex to grasp, especially since we've been conditioned to believe that emotions are purely neurological.

Let's explore an intriguing scientific study that challenges this perspective. In 1980, neurologist John Lorber reported on a student with severe hydrocephalus (water on the brain). The student was referred to him because he had an unusually large head. The findings were that the student's brain was compressed to a thin layer lining the skull, occupying only about 5% of the cranial cavity. So basically, he mainly had water in his head, not brain tissue. Remarkably, this individual had an IQ of 126 and earned a first-class honours degree in mathematics, demonstrating high cognitive function despite the minimal brain tissue (Lorber, 1980). If you look on YouTube, you will see similar stories. What does this mean? It suggests that emotions, memories, intelligence, creativity and the essence of who you are can be stored and processed beyond just the brain.

If emotions aren't confined to the brain, where else might they be? Some research suggests that emotions can be stored in different body parts — trapped in our muscles, organs, or energetic fields. Have you ever experienced an emotional release during a deep tissue massage or felt a wave of grief come out of nowhere? It's as if the body remembers. And what if it's not just the body? Could our emotions also be held in The *Field* — that invisible, energetic web connecting everything? Absolutely!

In addition to Austin's research, many other studies discuss how water can hold information and its connection to consciousness. One example is the book *The Hidden Messages of Water* by Japanese scientist Dr. Masaru Emoto. If you want to dive deeply into water and consciousness, start with these two recommended authors.

The idea that water, even tears, can store and carry energetic imprints of information offers a profound perspective on the act of crying. If tears hold traces of our emotions, then each drop becomes a tangible way to release what's been weighing us down — physically and energetically. Far from mere 'leaks,' tears are like tiny vessels of healing, reminding us that crying isn't just an emotional response but a profoundly transformative process, cleansing the heart and soul in poetic and scientific ways.

So, the next time you feel those tears welling up, don't fight it; crying isn't a sign of weakness. It's your body's way of hitting the reset button, healing old wounds, and clearing the path for whatever's next. In the words of Veider Austin (and perhaps your inner knowing), let it flow — let it heal.

My Final Words on Emotions. Many call this step of releasing emotions shadow work; whatever we name it, you must find a balance. Some people barely touch the sides, meaning they see a trapped emotion and then move on, thinking that just acknowledging it for a moment is enough. On the flip side, others take it too far, where shadow work becomes their whole life. When they constantly fixate on that emotion and their 'story', they continue to live in its frequency. It's not healthy to make shadow work your whole existence. Why? Because you may become a little self-absorbed. There are even some hardcore teachings out there that want you to feel no pain ever, to dissociate from everything, no matter what you are presented with. It's all about balance.

We are here in our bodies to experience the wondrous human life, full of love and pain, and we don't want to be completely numb; that's a bit of a dull existence. I believe feeling and experiencing emotions is part of being human, so don't beat yourself up if you feel emotions. We mentioned spiritual bypassing in the introduction; we can't skip the basic steps, but we also can't take it too far. There needs to be a balance with everything, so if you feel like you are engulfing your life with this work, take a step back, have a break, and be human for a while.

Keep checking in with yourself, and remember, not all emotions are hidden in the depths of you. Look at anxiety: it shows you very loudly that it's here. Pay attention to what you are doing or thinking when negative emotions or anxiety hit. Instead of pushing it down or numbing it, be aware and follow the steps. Along the way, always be kind to yourself.

Important Notes

1. I want to acknowledge that I don't know where you are with your emotions or how deep or significant your wounds might be. Please be kind to yourself and seek help if needed. If things feel overwhelming or you're dealing with deep trauma, it's okay to pause. Forget the tools and self-assessments for now; simply drop into your heart. Breathe through your heart, focus on it, feel it, and elevate your emotions toward love. Chapter 2 has more on heart coherence if you need to revisit it. This simple practice can work wonders, especially if you're frazzled and unsure what to do next. And remember, if you feel you need one-on-one professional support, seek it. Be careful who you work with; you don't want to go over your story for years; you want to move on.

2. I've noticed an interesting shift in the world. In my generation and older, many people suppressed their emotions and put on a happy face. In contrast, some younger generations today do the opposite, openly sharing their traumas, sometimes making it their identity. While it's vital to acknowledge your pain, there's a balance to be found. Admit to yourself that you have some emotional patterns to work through, but don't let them define your life. It's okay to share with trusted loved ones, but the whole world doesn't need to know every detail unless your story genuinely serves to help others. Before sharing, take a moment to check in with your ego. Be honest: Are you seeking validation or attention or genuinely sharing to inspire and uplift? If you realise you are doing it for attention, it's time to say, 'Enough of the woe is me; I'm going to change my frequency and move towards love'. Guess what? The more love you give, the more you get in return.

Before we close this chapter, ask yourself: *Will you continue living as the version of yourself shaped by fear and limitation, or are you ready to step into the full power of your heart—the radiant, limitless essence of who you truly are?* Your shadows are not here to define you; they are here to guide you. Within each one lies a gift, waiting to awaken your inner light.

Thank you for getting through that heavy topic. Let's recap the book up until this point because I know we've covered a lot. We've explored *the Field* and heart coherence (the heart is everything, by the way). Through self-exploration, we explored who we are, examined the shadows we may be hiding or ignoring, and learnt ways to release them. There will be more on releasing emotions in the meditation chapter.

Hopefully, you've gained some powerful tools and are excited about your new life. But trust me, we haven't reached the really fun stuff yet.
Next, we'll tackle Step 3, clearing our bridges by reshaping our thinking and rewiring our old, outdated programs.

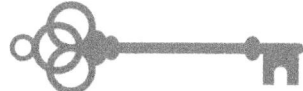

When I release my shadows, I bring light in.

CHAPTER 5

THOUGHT SCULPTING

STEP 3

Reprogram the way you think – like a Mental Makeover.

It's Time to Change That Programming

The last chapter was a bit heavy; after all, emotions are the messy masterpieces of human existence. Let's change the channel and dive into the quirks, habits, and stories that make us hilariously human. I want you to have fun with this chapter and laugh at yourself when you encounter some of your programming.

What is thought sculpting? Visualise thought sculpting as if you are an artist shaping clay; your mind is the medium, and your life is the creation. This chapter introduces how you can consciously rewire your thoughts, taking old crusty beliefs and reshaping them into something empowering and fresh. Think of it as upgrading from a worn-out VHS tape to high-definition streaming — wait, are you even old enough to know what a VHS tape is? If not, imagine buffering internet, which is as equally painful! Sure, it's hard work, but with each chip, you're rewiring your inner dialogue and creating a brand-new narrative. Fun right? (Okay, maybe not *fun* like eating chocolate cake, but you get the point!)

As we've explored in earlier chapters, thoughts are powerful. They're like invisible Wi-Fi signals carrying information, syncing with the world around you and influencing your outer reality in ways you might not even realise. Just as we've learned that emotions are energy in motion, thoughts are energy infused with information — but there is a difference. Positive emotions help you broadcast into the Field, while your thoughts act as the signal, directing that information toward what you desire. Think of it like this: positive emotions are like the key that unlocks the door to *the Field*, but your thoughts decide where that door leads you. The Field is magnetic and will offer a world that matches your thoughts and feelings. Changing your emotions and thoughts is helpful as we move into this book's meditation and manifesting sections. Trying to create a new reality while those old, poorly programmed thoughts still run in the background is like playing a beautiful symphony on a piano with broken keys. Sure, you might produce a few good notes, but imagine how much easier and more harmonious it will be when your mind and emotions are synchronised and coherent. We cannot change our outer world until we create the space to do so. If we continue operating solely from our conditioned programming, there is no room for free will or transformation. Instead, we remain trapped in the repetitive loops of our programmed minds. Remember, most of our thoughts aren't even true.

Just as we learn to pay attention to our emotions when triggered in a particular moment, the same principle applies to our thoughts. The beauty of thought sculpting lies in its intentionality — catching a runaway thought mid-pattern, rolling up your sleeves, and sculpting it into something you want. It's the mental equivalent of yelling, *'Opposite World!'* in your head. However, let's be honest: if you shouted it out loud every time, people might start looking at you in a funny way, or worse, they might lock you up. Still, it *would* be entertaining!

Picture this: you're stuck in traffic and your mind spirals. 'Great, I'm going to be late. My boss will think I'm unreliable, which is exactly why my life is a mess.' Now pause. Here's your chance to sculpt. You grab that thought by the tail and reshape it, 'Okay, I'm in traffic, but I can't control it. Let me use this time to listen to a podcast or brainstorm for my big idea.' Boom! You've just stepped one foot into *Opposite World,* where your best self hangs out, sipping tea and casually crushing it at life. And who knows? With your new thoughts and elevated frequency, the traffic might start clearing up, too.

Another example: Many of us habitually focus on what's lacking. Do any of these ring a bell?

> 'They never appreciate me.'
> 'I could never afford that.'
> 'I'm always late.'
> 'I'll never find someone who understands me.'

Hmmm, are these your affirmations?

What if, instead, you sculpt those thoughts into something like these:

'I'm grateful for the times they do show me appreciation.'

'I will be able to afford that soon.'

'I am not going to be late anymore.'

'I'm learning to understand myself better, which will naturally attract someone who aligns with me.'

Regularly practising these shifts of gratitude and abundance-focused thinking can become your *natural* way of seeing the world. Instead of constantly seeing the glass as half-empty, you'll train your brain always to see it as half-full. Remember the chapter on heart coherence? Living from your heart can instantly change your thoughts and the energy around you. Here's a little tip: if you struggle to escape a chain of negative thoughts, ask yourself: **What would love do?**

When confronted with a challenge, we all know someone who immediately jumps to what could go wrong or why it wouldn't work. Maybe that someone is you. But can you imagine if your *default* response was to think of what could go *right*? What if your natural state automatically gravitated toward optimism and possibility instead of doubt and fear? Here's the good news: You can rewire this. Thought sculpting gives you the tools to take control. Depending on your programs, it could be a quick tweak or take months of practice. Keep chipping away at those old patterns, and resculpt every time you notice a negative thought. Over time, your masterpiece, the new empowered you, will emerge.

I want to share an example of what our thoughts can create. We discussed emotions and our health in the previous chapter.

Let's also look at the power of our thoughts — the mirror that the universe can create. Many years ago, when I wasn't as in tune with my body, I started experiencing strange symptoms, like tingling down one side of my body and other odd sensations. The symptoms became so severe that I ended up in the hospital. The doctors referred me to a neurologist because they believed I might have multiple sclerosis (MS) based on my symptoms. Hearing those words completely freaked me out, and I had to wait weeks to see the specialist.

I went home and began researching my symptoms online. No kidding — within days, I had developed almost every symptom I had read about. I ended up bedridden for a week, convinced I had this illness. Fast forward to my appointment: after brain scans and further tests, it turned out I didn't have MS at all. Surprise, surprise, the symptoms vanished almost immediately.

Looking back, I realise my belief system had created those symptoms. My fear and focus on the disease allowed my mind to amplify and manifest the very symptoms I feared. Many years later, I came to believe that the original symptoms may have been caused by aspartame, the artificial sweetener in Diet Coke. At the time, I was drinking it daily, under the illusion that calorie counting meant you were healthy (programming), without understanding the harmful chemicals I was consuming. I will add that I no longer count calories but instead watch chemicals. I mention that because in *Opposite World*, we research everything, not just follow fads around like sheep. I tell this story to show how powerful our thoughts can be, but we can use this information to create superpowers.

Let's look at another example. Meet Summer, a talented graphic designer who dreaded client presentations. Every time she prepared to pitch her work, the same thought loop played: *'What if they think it's terrible? I'm not talented enough.'* Her work was good, but she found it hard to believe in herself. One day, a mentor introduced her to thought sculpting and how to change her energy.

Instead of letting her mind run wild with self-doubt, Summer worked hard to nail her next presentation. She began catching her negative thoughts as if they were raw clay blocks. Summer would pause, take a deep breath, and intentionally reshape them into something empowering. When it was time for her presentation, she changed her inner dialogue: *'They will love it. I've worked hard, and my designs add value.'*

Summer knew it wasn't just about changing her thoughts but also about elevating her emotions. Summer paired her new thoughts with gratitude and excitement, knowing these high-energy emotions carried powerful signals to *the Field*. She wasn't faking these thoughts and feelings; she was genuinely excited for the new person she was becoming internally. For the first time, she had created a ripple of confidence that extended beyond her.

When she gave her next presentation, something incredible happened. Not only did she feel more self-assured, but her clients also seemed more engaged and enthusiastic. By changing her energy, Summer noticed she had shifted the energy in the room. Her clients left inspired and asked her to lead their next big project.

Summer realised that thought sculpting wasn't just about silencing self-doubt. It was also about believing her new thoughts, feeling the emotions of her expected outcomes and creating a new reality. Whenever doubt crept in, she'd remind herself: *'I'm the sculptor, not the clay. My thoughts create my reality.'* She realised she was the creator of her life.

Thought–Emotion Loop

Earlier, we touched on how emotions tune you into the frequency of the Field while your thoughts act as the signal, directing that energy toward what you desire. But what happens when your emotions and thoughts create a loop, feeding off each other in ways that might not always work in your favour?

This loop is like a two-way street. A negative thought can trigger a low-vibration emotion, such as fear, frustration or sadness. That emotion, in turn, amplifies the original thought, making it feel more challenging to escape. It's a feedback loop, cycling endlessly and keeping you stuck in the same patterns. For example, a thought like 'I'll never be good at this' can evoke feelings of defeat, reinforcing similar thoughts like 'Why even try?' Of course, if you say you will never be good at something, the Field will grant that wish. Remember, your life mirrors your thoughts, emotions and beliefs, so be careful what you say and think.

But here's the empowering part: just as the loop can keep you stuck, it can also be a powerful tool for change. You can interrupt the loop by shifting your thoughts and elevating your emotions. This hack will completely transform the energy you're putting into the Field. Imagine catching a negative thought and reshaping it. When you break the cycle, you stop being a prisoner to your old programming. Instead, you take charge of your mind and emotions, steering them toward a reality you want to create.

If all this talk of sculpting your thoughts feels overwhelming, and you think, '*Opposite World* sounds like hard work,' let me tell you: It doesn't have to be so daunting. Next, I will offer some suggestions to help it feel more manageable.

Stepping into Neutrality: A Booster Step

You may find that changing a thought to the opposite is just too big a step, and you know you won't believe it at a deep level. What if we made it easier? Take the middle road and step into neutrality first. So instead of saying, 'I am going to be amazing at this', say something like, 'This is challenging, but I'm learning.' That slight shift changes the thought and triggers a new emotional response, like curiosity or determination, which feeds into even better thoughts.

Instead of trying to leap from negative to positive in one giant jump, we can take a gentler step in between. Sometimes, the gap between negativity and positivity feels like an unbridgeable canyon, but here's the secret: there's a perfect bridge we can call Neutrality. Also remind yourself to take a neutral break in the middle if it feels too much of a stretch. It's like a booster step; this mindset can be used in anything we do when heading to *Opposite World*. At least then, you will still be putting out a higher frequency to the Field than if you remained with the same negative thoughts.

Neutrality is your stepping stone, a safe and manageable middle ground. When your thoughts are profoundly negative, they might feel fake or forced to shift into gratitude or joy immediately. For example, if your thoughts are 'Everything is falling apart', it's hard to believe something like, 'Life is amazing!' Instead, neutrality invites you to pause and acknowledge the situation without judgment. A better way to approach your thoughts would be: 'Things aren't going as planned right now, but that doesn't mean they'll stay this way forever.'

Neutrality is about smoothing out the jagged edges of your thought patterns before you try to sculpt something new. It's like clearing a messy workspace before starting a masterpiece. By choosing neutral, nonjudgmental thoughts, you stop fuelling negative emotions and create space for something better. For instance, if you think, 'I always mess things up,' you can shift to, 'I'm learning as I go.' It's not overly optimistic, but it's not destructive either — it's just true.

From this place of neutrality, taking the next step toward positive, empowering thoughts becomes much more manageable. It's like finding a calm clearing in the middle of a storm; once you're there, you can decide how to move forward with clarity and intention. I do speak with experience of this working. Quite a few years ago, I was in a situation where my life was really bad; people couldn't understand why I wasn't in a negative spin, rocking in a corner. I was very blessed that my emotions were relatively high because my thoughts kept telling me, 'Well, this is kind of exciting because if things are this bad now, only good things will come, eventually.' I didn't know about the principle of polarity then, but it was a great example of how our thinking can help us in trauma or stressful situations. We will discuss the principle of polarity shortly, but keep this example in mind because we will flip the way you think.

In the following section, I have compiled several tools you can use when you catch yourself reverting to old ways. You can use one or all of them. Before we look at those, let's examine typical human behaviour and how you can think differently.

Chipping Away

As well as using the neutrality step to bridge your thought-changing process, remember that thought sculpting is about chipping away slowly, intentionally, and with patience. Just like an artist shaping a block of marble or a caterpillar transforming into a butterfly, this is not an overnight process. Each time you catch and reshape a negative thought, you remove a tiny piece of the old, unhelpful pattern and reveal something new and beautiful underneath. It may feel subtle initially, but those small, consistent shifts create lasting transformation. You may have 100 negative thoughts over the day and manage to convert two — this is a successful day. People are hard on themselves when doing this work and expect instant changes. Just keep saying to yourself, I am chipping away. These programmes have been there for a very long time, so be patient with yourself. Over time, accumulating these micro-changes will unveil a whole new version of your inner world — true, lasting change happens gradually, with persistence and grace. So be kind and gentle with yourself and surrender to love.

Does this sound easier? Because we want you in *Opposite World*. The fact that you're reading this book means it's precisely where you're meant to be.

The Daily Thought-Sculpting Game

Let's make thought sculpting so easy and playful that it feels like a game, a fun challenge you look forward to each day. Here's a tool you can use right now to bring creativity and joy into the process.

1. **Name your inner sculptor** First, give your inner thought sculptor a fun, quirky name. A name that makes you smile. Maybe it's 'Chisel Charlie,' 'Cosmic Artist', 'Sculpting Sylvia', or you could call it 'Fred'. The idea is to personify this part of you so it feels like you've got a friendly companion helping you catch and reshape those thoughts.

2. **Spot and sculpt** Each day, challenge yourself to catch three negative or limiting thoughts. When you notice one, pause and say (out loud or in your head), 'Hey, [insert your sculptor's name], let's reshape this!' This playful interruption makes the process less severe and helps you engage creatively. Each time you catch a negative thought, ask yourself, 'Is that the affirmation I want to put in the Field?'

   Some examples:

- Negative thought: 'I always mess this up.'
- Sculpted thought: 'I'm figuring this out, and each step gets me closer.'
- Negative thought: 'I can't afford that.'
- Sculpted thought: 'I am putting the actions in place and will get that.'

3. **The Opposite World Flip** When you catch a negative thought, imagine stepping into *Opposite World*, where your best, most empowered self lives. You could even give yourself a new name in *Opposite World*, like Hercules. Ask yourself, 'What would [...] think'? For instance, if your thought is, 'This is too hard', your positive side in *Opposite World* might think, 'I love challenges — they make me stronger.'

Some people like to use a word when they catch that pesky Mr/Mrs Negative, like 'change' or 'stop' or 'go away, Mr Nego' or whatever works for you.

4. **Keep Score** If negative thoughts are your life's nemesis, turn them into a game by keeping track of how many thoughts you sculpt each day. Reward yourself when you reach a certain number. The goal isn't perfection; it's progress. Each thought you reshape is a small win!

5. **Nightly Reflection** Before bed, take a moment to reflect on the thoughts you sculpted that day. Celebrate your wins, no matter how small. You could even keep a journal to jot down your original thoughts and their sculpted versions, creating a record of your transformation over time. It's like having a gallery of your mental masterpieces.

~

For those who are already naturally wired to think positively, amazing! You can skip the steps above, but take a moment to appreciate how your thoughts transpire in your life. Recognise the power of your positive mental wiring and how it creates opportunities, connections, and joy. Of course, we're all human, and Mr or Mrs Nego (that pesky voice of negativity) will visit now and then. The goal isn't to banish him/her entirely but to ensure that your thoughts usually reflect the positive, empowering frequency that helps you thrive.

Important Note:

I want to make a point that may help you find peace. Not every thought you have will create noticeable changes in your life. Why? For a thought to truly take root and influence your reality, it must carry energy — meaning, it must be backed by feelings or emotions.

Let me give you an example: Your days are mostly wired with negative undertones. Imagine you've just spilled coffee on your favourite shirt and, while muttering about your day is terrible, you try to slap a cheerful thought on top like, *'But at least I have coffee!'* yet you still feel annoyed and frustrated. That positive thought doesn't stand a chance against the emotional storm underneath!

On the contrary, if your inner dialogue is primarily positive but you have a fleeting negative thought, like, *'What if I mess this up?'* Don't worry; it's not going to stick. Why? Because your emotions behind it are still rooted in positivity and confidence, which are far stronger forces.

In the previous chapter, we explored the importance of emotions, but this point bears repeating. While your thoughts send the information, your feelings amplify and anchor them; they are the energetic carriers. When the two are aligned, they create the resonance that shapes your experiences. This knowledge will be worth knowing when we get to the manifestation chapter.

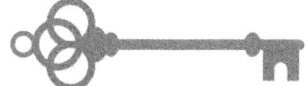

The thoughts I choose to focus on shape the life I create.

The Principles of Polarity – Think to the Opposite

What if I told you that every problem you face already holds its solution, hidden in plain sight, like two sides of the same coin, inseparable and waiting for you to flip your perspective? I want to introduce you to a universal truth: the principles of polarity. This ancient principle is the biggest plot twist in the book so far. Why? So far, we have focused on doing, thinking, and feeling the opposite of what we've been conditioned to do in our old patterns. But here comes that twist: once you've fully stepped into *Opposite World* and made it your home, it's no longer opposite; it becomes your natural state. That revelation brings us to *the principles of polarity, which is a* profound principle that will challenge how you see duality, contrast, and transformation in your life. Earlier in this chapter, I touched on this principle and shared how, during a crisis, my natural response was to believe that if things were this bad, something great had to be on the horizon — almost to the point of excitement. It wasn't until years later that I realised this mindset was more than optimism; it was a built-in coping mechanism.

What is polarity? In straightforward terms, Polarity is the idea that everything has two opposite sides or extremes, but they are actually connected and part of the same thing. Another description could be that polarity teaches us that opposites are not separate but are two ends of the same spectrum, and one cannot exist without the other.

What are the principles of polarity, and where do they originate? I first studied the principle of polarity in The Kybalion, it was written in 1908 by three anonymous authors under the pseudonym 'The Three Initiates'. They took ancient teachings and put them into practical principles for the modern age. The principle of polarity is one of the seven Hermetic principles outlined in The Kybalion. The original teachings were attributed to Hermes Trismegistus, a legendary figure who was said to embody the wisdom of the Greek god Hermes and the Egyptian god Thoth. While the exact origins of these teachings remain mysterious, their roots stretch back thousands of years to ancient Egypt, where Thoth was revered as the god of wisdom and writing.

Hermetic texts are a fusion of Egyptian and Greek wisdom created during the Hellenistic period (roughly 1st–3rd centuries CE). These writings include philosophical, mystical, and practical teachings about the nature of reality, the divine, the soul, alchemy, and the cosmos. I encourage you to read The Kybalion; it has such profound messages about life.

The principle of polarity teaches us that opposites are merely extremes of the same thing — love and hate, hot and cold, light and dark. The description of the principle of polarity is 'the all and the many are the same,' meaning that opposites are not truly separate but are simply different degrees of the same essence.

Let's look at some examples: Love and hate may seem like opposites, but they exist on the same emotional spectrum. Imagine a couple who just broke up. Furious and heartbroken, one partner exclaims, 'I hate them!' But do they really? Hate, after all, is just love wearing its darkest disguise. The depth of their anger comes from the depth of their love, love flipped inside out. If they truly didn't care, indifference would have taken the stage. Love and hate are two sides of the same coin, dancing on the spectrum of passion. Hermetic teachings state that the middle point of love and hate is like and dislike, which gradually shade into each other and become a point we can't distinguish between. *The Kybalion* states that you can transform hate into love by using your will (Three Initiates, 1908). This concept is complex and challenging to get your head around, but keep working on it. Of course, hate isn't always twisted love; it can also arise from deep wounds, betrayal, or injustice. Hate is an energy that holds power over us until it transforms. The path to that transformation often involves forgiveness, which we'll dive into later.

Other examples explaining the principle of polarity are hot and cold; these are merely different points on the temperature scale. Or think about electricity; it depends on the interplay of positive and negative charges. The principle of polarity teaches us that these opposites are necessary to create balance, growth, and transformation in our lives. *The Kybalion* is an excellent starting point if you'd like to explore this concept further.

Why learn the principles of polarity? Because understanding that every situation exists on a spectrum allows us to add calmness to a chaotic world. It helps us recognise that challenges and growth, joy and pain, light and dark, are different degrees of the same thing. Think of this knowledge as a powerful tool in your belt, allowing you to shift your experience along the scale rather than being stuck at one extreme. This understanding is like having next-level resilience.

Here's a practical example: Imagine you're feeling stressed, your heart is racing, your mind is spinning, and everything feels overwhelming. Instead of thinking, 'I need to calm down' (which can feel like an impossible leap), you use the principle of polarity to recognise that calmness and stress exist on the same emotional spectrum. Stress isn't the opposite of calm; it's a heightened state of the same energy. By consciously choosing to slow your breathing or take a slight pause, you're not trying to leap into calmness; you're simply shifting your position slightly down the scale. You could visualise it like turning down a dial. As you practice, you notice that stress can transform into focus, and focus can naturally evolve into calm.

The principle of polarity teaches us to work with the spectrum rather than resist one end. This understanding helps us see that we don't need to fight or escape what we're feeling; we need to nudge it toward a more desirable state, step by step. The beauty of this principle lies in its simplicity: when you can see that light and dark, love and fear, or even success and failure are all connected, you can move with life's natural rhythms instead of resisting them.

We can utilise the principle of polarity when practising our thought sculpting, as it teaches us that every challenge carries its opposite solution, like two ends of the same rope. When sculpting your thoughts, you pull that rope toward the reality you want to create. Take Maya, for example. After a tough breakup, she found herself stuck in a negative headspace with thoughts like, *'I'll never find love again,'* feeling emotions of sadness and rejection. But as she started sculpting her thoughts, she realised the breakup wasn't the end of life as she knew it; it was the beginning of rediscovering her worth. She shifted her focus to thoughts like, *'This is my chance to build the life I truly want,'* and paired those thoughts with feelings of hope and self-love. Slowly, her energy began to change. She felt lighter, and her newfound confidence began attracting healthier relationships and opportunities. When you mindfully sculpt your thoughts like Maya, you're not just escaping the pain but transforming it. By shifting to the complementary side of polarity, you create the space to align with your highest potential and write a new chapter for yourself.

Visual Tool: When life feels overwhelming, remind yourself: 'It's all the same energy. I need to adjust the dial.' Picture a light dimmer or a volume knob and imagine yourself turning it slightly to shift your experience to a more manageable level. It's not about jumping to the opposite extreme; it's about tweaking the energy just enough to regain balance.

Suppose you have managed to grasp this way of thinking. Well done! It's a difficult one to get your head around. Many may think you've just heard another language from another planet, but sit with it and study it. Learning this principle can seriously change things in your life. You don't just magically grasp concepts like this; it actually takes work.

Everything is dual; everything has poles; everything has its pair of opposites; like and unlike are the same; opposites are identical in nature but different in degree; extremes meet; all truths are but half-truths; all paradoxes may be reconciled.

– Extract from *The Kybalion*

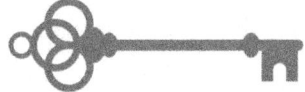

Suffering fades when I recognise the polarity within it.

CHAPTER 6

BE YOUR ALCHEMIST FOR TRANSFORMATION

STEP 4

It's time to create some magic.

What is Alchemy?

Becoming an Alchemist is our final step in clearing our bridge. Our first step was getting to know ourselves on a deeper level (self-awareness); then we looked at our shadows within (emotions); next, we learnt about our thoughts (programming/mindset); and now, I like to call this final step: how to bring out the magician in us (transformation). What is alchemy? Traditionally, alchemy was the ancient practice of transforming base metals, like lead, into gold. But beyond its literal meaning, alchemy has always symbolised something deeper, the process of profound transformation and mastery over the self. It's about taking something ordinary, even undesirable, and turning it into something extraordinary.

Now, what does it mean to be your own alchemist? It means taking the tools and insights you've gathered so far and using them to transform your inner world and transmute your energies. You've explored who you are, identified the patterns that no longer serve you, and learnt how to shift your thoughts and emotions. It's time to create some magic. Alchemy is the next step: it's the process of consciously creating your new reality. It's about recognising your ability to take the 'raw material' of your current life, no matter how messy, challenging, or incomplete it may feel, and refine it into something brilliant, meaningful, and uniquely yours.

Why is this the next step in our journey? Because transformation begins within. Everything we've covered so far — understanding who you are, learning how to navigate emotions and thoughts, and stepping into the energy of change — has prepared you for this moment. So, if you are not ready to create some magic, go back over the previous chapters and spend more time with them. There is no rush — do this at your own pace.

You are equipped to become the creator of your own life, turning challenges into opportunities and intentions into tangible outcomes. In *Opposite World*, you're not just living differently; you're crafting a new masterpiece with every choice, thought, and action.

Changing Patterns

We can all be our own alchemists and rewire our subconscious, transforming the energy that shapes our reality. As we've discussed, most programming sits quietly in the subconscious, influencing our thoughts, behaviours, and decisions without us even realising it. Guess what? A lot of this programming isn't even true! Let's look at some proof of this.

Several research studies show that much of what we remember is not accurate. For example, in a study conducted in 2002, 20 participants were exposed to a fabricated childhood event. They did this by showing a doctored photograph depicting them on a hot-air balloon ride. During three interviews, 50% of these participants developed complete or partial false memories of the event (Wade et al., 2002). So, let go of all the stories that don't serve you because there is a big chance that they are inaccurate.

We've already explored how patterns appear in different areas of our lives, and now it's time to go deeper. Think of your subconscious programming as an outdated computer system downloaded long ago and full of glitches and inaccuracies. As we are learning, many of the stories we carry around aren't even based on fact. Yet, because they're stored in the 'back office' of our minds, we accept them as truth. Our beliefs quietly dictate our reality; we usually don't question or update them. Why don't we do audits on our beliefs? We must keep up to date in our careers and other areas of life. Humans are creatures of habit, often sticking to the same way of thinking day in day out. But newsflash: the world evolves, perspectives shift, and countless other beliefs exist. What makes yours the ultimate truth? Maybe it's time for an upgrade.

Power of Forgiveness

We've discussed the need to face our shadows head-on for our health (both physical and mental). Although I would love to explore every emotion, this book could not fit them all in. I would, however, like to discuss the power of forgiveness. I introduced this earlier when talking about the emotion of hate in the principles of polarity. We are told not to hold grudges and to let them go; there is some deep reasoning behind this. Many people I have talked to who have experienced emotional or physical healing have said their journey began with forgiveness. I can also attest to this powerful shift. Transmuting resentment into forgiveness can heal you neurologically, physically, and spiritually. Let's look at these.

Neurobiological – A little science here; bear with me. Studies have shown that forgiveness can change brain waves (John Hopkins Medicine, 2024). Forgiveness impacts physical and mental health, including stress reduction and emotional regulation, which are connected to changes in brain waves, particularly in emotional regulation and empathy areas. Studies suggest that practising forgiveness can:
- Calm the amygdala (part of the brain that controls and stores emotions)
- Reduce negative emotions and strengthen the prefrontal cortex (the thinking part of the brain that handles decision-making and planning)
- Enhancing decision-making and emotional control.

Consider this: if these changes happen in the brain when you forgive, what happens to it when you are holding grudges? You are probably stuck in fight-or-flight mode (remember how stress affects your health!) and may also be experiencing brain fog. These are your mind's way of begging you to let go.

Body Health — Forgiveness could lead to lower stress levels, improved mental clarity, reduced anxiety, and better overall well-being (Worthington & Scherer, 2004). It also contributes to lower blood pressure and improved sleep quality. Forgiveness has been known to help with conditions like vertigo and even increase endurance. Forgiveness is also your step towards heart coherence.

Spirituality — Many spiritual traditions view forgiveness as a transformative practice. It is thought to heal and offer inner peace and emotional freedom, like unburdening the soul. Forgiveness can transcend space and time and change frequencies with the person you are forgiving, perhaps even putting them on a path to awakening.

There are teachings from the Christian Bible about forgiveness. It teaches believers to practice forgiveness as a continual, transformative process.

Then Peter came to Jesus and asked, 'Lord, how many times shall I forgive my brother or sister who sins against me? Up to seven times?' Jesus answered, 'I tell you, not seven times, but seventy-seven times'. (Matthew 18:21-22.)

Forgiveness in Buddhism is linked to the law of karma. By forgiving, individuals release themselves from the karmic consequences of holding onto negative emotions like anger or hatred.

∼

In *Opposite World*, we learn to forgive because the flip side of forgiveness will release the burden on your body and mind. Forgiveness does not mean you have to reconcile with the person who has done you wrong, nor does it condone what they have done. It also doesn't mean you don't seek justice if their actions are illegal. It is more of a selfish act: why would you want to have health issues brought on by a person who has done wrong to you; why would you want shadows left in your body from them? So please think about whether you are holding any resentment toward someone and use the letting go tool in Chapter 4 to alchemise that emotion. It may take a day, a month or a year, but slowly work on it and then pay attention to any difference in your physical, mental and spiritual self.

Let go of the story; it's not your story anymore. Leave the burden with them. It's time to alchemise your resentment by transmuting it with love into empathy, sympathy, compassion, and especially love. Please do this — do it for yourself. Always remember that only love can heal. This will take back your power — you deserve that.

Alchemy: Transmuting Fear into Love

If the idea of alchemy is about turning the ordinary into the extraordinary, then the ultimate creation is turning fear into love. From an internal perspective, fear is often considered the root of all negative emotions. Think of fear as being food for all lower frequencies. If you delve deep enough into any uncomfortable feeling, you will often find fear sitting at the core. For instance, feelings of unworthiness might stem from a fear of rejection or not being good enough. By continually asking yourself, 'Why? Why do I feel this way? Why does it matter?' you will gradually uncover fear is the root of your emotions. At the very bottom layer, this fear often boils down to the fear of death, whether it is a physical, emotional, or symbolic death.

When fear takes over, it can feel like this:

F - F@#*k

E- Everything

A - And

R- Run

We've all been there—overwhelmed, panicked, and ready to escape at the first sign of discomfort.

But what if fear isn't what it seems?

F- False

E- Expectations

A- Appearing

R- Real

Most fears are based on imagined worst-case scenarios. When we recognise this, we reclaim our power.

The choice is yours: Will fear control you, or will you see it for what it is?

If you want to simplify your emotions, consider that there are only two: fear and love. Every other emotion is just a word. That way, when trying to dissolve emotions, you can think of them as fear being alchemised into love.

Fear needs to be tackled head-on; otherwise, your only experience with what you fear will remain negative. Fear disrupts our connection to oneness and the frequency of the Field. There are so many distractions in society that keep us in fear. People hold on to fear because they think it keeps them safe, but love keeps them safe. Fear is a contracted force stuck inside us, whereas love is expansive; it is everywhere. We can learn to love and heal our bodies when we are free of fear.

The more you avoid something you fear, the worse it will get. Let's look at an example of a type of fear: phobias. Phobias may be easy to tackle because they appear very clearly in your external world. So be the master and challenge your fears. Of course, as long as the fears are not dangerous, you don't need to chase lions. Let's take a simple example: say you have an irrational fear of lizards. Imagine gently holding one in your hand, reminding yourself that it's a part of you, just as you are a part of it. As we've explored, we are all connected, and this connection can foster compassion for something as small as Mr Lizard. If that feels like too big a step at first, start small, get close to it, observe it, and gradually work toward holding it. With time, love, and consistency, what was once a source of fear can become an experience of understanding and even connection. Transmute that fear to love, and who knows, you may end up with a pet lizard.

So, we've mentioned LOVE many times, and since we want to alchemise our emotions to love, let's talk about it — what is love? If the Field is the infinite source of connection and possibilities, then love is the energy that moves through it, binding everything together; it is the material of the universe. Love isn't just a fleeting emotion; it's a state of being that transforms how we see the world and ourselves. Allowing love to guide us can shift our outlook entirely, dissolving fear and softening the edges of negative emotions.

Being in a state of love is like switching on a light in a dark room; it illuminates what was hidden, brings clarity, and makes everything feel a little less overwhelming. In those moments of fear, anger, or doubt, a simple question can bring you back to the centre: *What would love do?* Love would choose compassion over judgment, courage over avoidance, and kindness over anger. Love is the absence of fear. It's not always the easiest choice, but it's the one that creates connection, healing, and growth.

And here in *Opposite World*, we're all about love, not just the easy kind but the kind that projects love even to people operating in much lower frequencies. Why? Because they're just stuck in their own 'normie world' bubble and don't even know *Opposite World* exists — yet. Love doesn't judge or push people away; it invites them in. So, if someone's negativity makes you want to run in the other direction, remember: Love's superpower is that it can exist even in the most challenging spaces. And maybe your love can be the spark that wakes someone in your life up to a new state of being.

We can use all the tools we've learnt to clear emotions and then shape our thoughts with the ultimate goal of love. Everything comes back to love. Living in your heart, in the feeling of love, is when actual creation happens. Love offers the space to create miracles, align with your higher self, and step fully into *Opposite World*. Love isn't just a feeling; it's the most powerful state of being and the key to transforming your inner and outer worlds.

If you would like to delve much deeper into this concept, *A Course in Miracles* offers profound insight into how this can be done spiritually. Written by psychologist Helen Schucman, who described the text as an 'inner dictation' from a voice she identified as Jesus, this long yet life-changing work guides readers toward profound transformation. Consisting of a text and a workbook, it's not for the faint of heart. Some find its depth overwhelming, choosing to focus solely on the workbook. But the rewards can be extraordinary for those who embark on the journey.

At its core, *A Course in Miracles* teaches that true inner peace and healing come through a shift in perception — from fear to love. This is where its teachings align beautifully with the concept of alchemy. Fear is like our minds 'base metal'; it is heavy and limiting. Love, on the other hand, is the 'gold' we are striving to create. The *Course* emphasises that miracles can only occur when the mind is free of fear. Through forgiveness, 'a key principle in the *Course*', we dissolve the illusions of separation and transform fear-based thinking into love-based awareness.

~

Let's look at alchemy from a straightforward perspective. If you want to eliminate an emotion, stop thinking about whatever it is and tune in to a different frequency. Say, for example, you have health anxiety, and you often fear getting sick. Just stop thinking about getting sick, change your frequency by being grateful for your good health and stay in the elevated emotions of gratitude and love. Remind yourself that disease exists in lower frequencies and fear is the food for these lower frequencies. Every time you slip back and have those looming thoughts, change them. By integrating these shifts of thoughts and emotions in our lives, we learn to live in alignment with love rather than fear, creating a more harmonious inner and outer reality. Following the steps in previous chapters of changing your thoughts and acknowledging stuck emotions, we can alchemise and shift these obstacles into love.

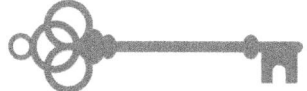

Miracles only happen when you choose love over fear.
—Course in Miracles

Flow State

As we've learnt, choosing love over fear is an act of alchemy that transforms our inner state and creates the foundation for something truly extraordinary. When we align with love and live in our hearts, we naturally release the resistance and chaos that fear creates. This opens the door to something extraordinary: *flow state*. Flow happens when we're fully present, effortlessly connected, and aligned with our highest potential. It's the state where creativity, focus, and joy thrive. In this state, we can alchemise our world much faster than trying to do it in our monkey brain. It's a place where life feels almost magical, and everything *clicks because you align with the Field*.

What is flow state? You may have heard it being referred to as 'Zen state', 'being in the zone', 'trance-like state', or endurance athletes may call it 'runners high'. Entering a flow state often involves reduced activity in the brain's prefrontal cortex, fully immersing people in the moment. I call it shutting down the monkey brain, which can sometimes drive you nuts. Let's take this frontal lobe offline or power it right down. Hopefully, you have found ways to calm the monkey with some of our previous exercises.

Reduced prefrontal cortex activity helps people let go of excessive self-monitoring and time awareness, creating that seamless, almost effortless focus often described as flow. It's one of the reasons people feel less inhibited, more intuitive, and able to absorb the task at hand. This flow state helps connect to the Field, aligning your mind and body with a natural, harmonious frequency. This state is ideal for working on your alchemy.

Sounds lovely, doesn't it? And it is. When you reach this state, time melts away; it feels like you are slipping into a gentle rhythm with the universe where each movement, thought, and breath feels perfectly aligned. In this state, connection to the Field feels effortless, almost like tapping into a hidden reservoir of energy and insight. There's a peaceful joy in knowing you're part of something bigger, and each moment flows into the next without hesitation. People often describe flow as a profound experience, like a union with something beyond themselves. It feels magical and becomes an effortless alignment. There is no time, just a being.

Here are some ways we can reach the flow state.

1. **Meditation** Regular meditation quiets the mind and creates the perfect conditions for flow. By silencing that inner monologue (the one that won't stop planning dinner while you're trying to focus), you can slip into a state of deep connection and clarity. The meditation chapter discusses this more.

2. **Breathwork** Techniques like the Wim Hof Method or rhythmic breathing can calm the nervous system. Think of it as hitting the 'reset' button for your brain and heart, syncing them into perfect harmony.

3. **Music and Sound** Music can be a powerful gateway to flow, whether binaural beats, isochronic tones, or blasting your

favourite playlist. We will discuss this further in Chapter 9, Meditation.

4. **Creative Outlets** Anything that puts you in a rhythm, such as painting, writing, gardening, or playing a musical instrument, can easily lead to flow, especially when you're so absorbed that you forget to check your phone (gasp!). Even doodling counts; yes, those stick figures are art!

5. **Nature Immersion** Whether hiking up a mountain or sitting on a park bench, spending time in nature connects you to the world's natural rhythms. Fresh air, chirping birds, the sound of a waterfall, watching fire and rain can all bring you into flow.

6. **Mindful Movement Practices** Yoga, tai chi, or qigong combine movement and breath to make your body feel like it is flowing to its internal soundtrack. Don't worry if you're not graceful; it's about syncing your mind and body.

7. **Journaling or Stream of Consciousness Writing** Letting your thoughts pour out onto paper without caring about grammar or whether they make sense can be surprisingly freeing. It's like giving your brain a coffee break while your hand takes over. And no one ever has to read it, so go wild! Some people also do automatic writing, which is like channelling from the Field.

8. **Connection with Animals** Spending mindful time with pets can bring you into flow. Animals live in the present moment, blissfully free of emails and existential crises. Our dogs love our meditation room because they sense the calm

energy there. Plus, studies show pets can sync their heart rhythms with yours. How's that for a man's best friend?

9. **Running, Dancing, or Other Exercise** Steady-paced activities like running, dancing, or any rhythmic exercise can create a meditative rhythm that naturally leads to flow. When your body moves harmoniously, your mind often follows, creating a sense of effortless focus and presence. Plus, it's a great way to boost your mood and energy!

10. **Plant Medicine** Some people explore flow state through plant medicines like mushrooms or ayahuasca, which have been used in spiritual and healing traditions for centuries. These substances can bring profound insights and help release deep-seated trauma, but they aren't for everyone and require careful guidance from a professional Sharman. Scientifically, these substances can alter blood flow in the brain, increasing it in regions associated with emotion and introspection and shifting blood away from areas related to constant mental chatter. Full caution must be taken on these stronger plants, and I wouldn't recommend them without experienced professionals, as they are not suited to certain people. For a gentler and more accessible plant medicine, you might explore reishi mushrooms or blue lotus flowers, which can help you ease into your flow state.

11. **Prayer** Prayer can be a powerful tool for entering a flow state. It involves setting clear intentions, surrendering control, and opening oneself to guidance or inspiration from a higher source. When practised with genuine emotion and trust, prayer can help one tap into a profound inner peace and flow state.

12. **Hypnosis** Hypnosis is a naturally occurring state of highly focused attention and deep relaxation in which the conscious mind becomes less active and the subconscious mind becomes more accessible. These states overlap. In a hypnosis state, it's possible to temporarily dissociate from overactive thoughts or mental blocks, allowing space for clarity, healing, and transformation. Hypnosis can help you release fears, uncover creative ideas, or reframe limiting beliefs, making it a powerful tool for achieving a flow state.

These activities can act as a portal to flow, whether through intense focus, rhythmic movement, or simply being fully present. The key is finding what resonates with you. Honestly, you can enter flow state even by doing the most mundane things in life, like washing the dishes. The more often we enter this trance-like state, the easier it becomes to rewire our minds. If you enter this state often, you will be more aware of synchronicities, messages in dreams, instincts and all the subtle cues you would usually dismiss. Once you've felt the magic of being in flow, you'll never forget it and never want to lose it. The key is always to remain open to its call.

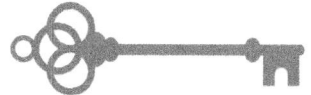

Surrender to allow flow.

Final Words on Alchemy

The magic of alchemy lies in your ability to transmute shadows through awareness, breath, and meditation. By bringing loving attention to these hidden parts of yourself, you can break old patterns, transforming your emotions, relationships, and even your health. Your shadows may simply be remnants of ancestral karma you've carried into this life—but instead of fearing them, embrace them as catalysts for growth and self-discovery.

Final Words on the Four Steps

That concludes our four steps to clear our bridge to the Field and our best life. Remember that your life is the mirror of your internal world. The way you think and see the world is based on your perceptions. Please pay attention to that voice in your head, the negative one, and know that it is not the real you. It is your programmed mind that thinks it is protecting you from harm. Fear-based programming will hold you back and limit your life. Don't be the person who says, 'It's just the way I am' — it's not; it's the way you have become. Another flaw to watch for is blaming outside reasons. Don't say, 'My life is like this because of … (outside reason)' — it's not; it's because of your internal world. Also, pay attention to your triggers; why did you react? Keep asking the questions. Instead of focusing on your problem/s and sitting in that frequency, turn it around to focus on solutions; this will create a whole new outer world for you. Self-awareness is like playing detectives with yourself, have fun with it and watch the changes.

Self-awareness is everything. Know that tiny daily changes make a big difference, so keep chipping away. We all have negative programming, and it would be impossible to be 100% clear of it (unless you are Buddha), but you can give it a beautiful cleanout. The more you understand yourself, the greater your life will be.

Remember not to let that programmed voice in your head hold you back. It holds all its information from past experiences, whether it was Johnny who dumped you, Mary who teased you, or your parents who expected perfection. Also, don't let other people control your emotions; you are the master of your emotions. So if you hear yourself say, 'he/she made me feel …' pull yourself up.

Step back, pay attention, watch yourself as if watching a movie, don't judge, be fascinated.

How do you know when you are starting to change?

When you intimately know yourself, when that fear-driven voice has faded, and you feel peace and joy. Your intuition will be sharp, and your inner world will feel calmer. You will handle situations better and be happier; what people say and do around you won't bother you. The negative voice will no longer be the director of your life. As you chip away at those thoughts and emotions that don't serve you, you will be closer to your higher self and the person you were meant to be. So, break free from these limiting beliefs and emotions, break free from the grip of your mind. Small changes made consistently give you big results. Always remember that love will guide you, and fear will restrict you.

Now, let's step away from this work for a while. Next, we will learn about the layers of the universe and our true selves and consider whether this is our only life.

CHAPTER 7

THE LAYERS OF YOU

Well done! You've completed the steps to clearing the bridge that leads you to your true self. We discussed entering a flow state, where we feel a profound sense of alignment that our mind, body, and spirit move together in perfect harmony. Time feels irrelevant, and everything flows effortlessly. It's like stepping into a better version of yourself. But how do we access that ease and alignment? The answer lies in understanding the layers of you.

We've encountered different terms throughout this book when discussing you, and although they are all deeply connected, they are not necessarily identical. What follows is a straightforward breakdown of your layers. Like the first chapter, The Field, this stuff can go very deep, but I'll keep it simple and easy to digest.

Your Body and Mind

Your physical body is your home base, the vehicle that allows your consciousness to interact with the world. The body exists in the third dimension (3D). It is here to help you feel, express, and heal. Without it, you wouldn't be able to taste chocolate or feel the sun's warmth on your skin. Think of it as the sturdy foundation that supports your journey of self-discovery. Later in the book, we have a chapter on ways to nourish the body. I will also explain 3D a bit further along.

Then there's the mind, paired with the ego, acting like a navigation system. What is the ego? Many people describe it differently, but in simple terms, the ego is the part of you that focuses on identity and self-preservation. It often keeps you tethered to fear, comparison, and a sense of separation. Interestingly, we innately recognise our oneness with everything when we are born. But over the first few years of life, we regress from this unity, gradually shifting into the perception of separateness, seeing ourselves as distinct from the world around us. This perception gives rise to the ego, a mechanism to help you navigate the world and feel safe.

If you've been following along, we've already gotten to know the mind quite well in the previous chapters — sometimes a little too well, am I right? It's great for getting through daily life but is often programmed by past experiences. Those old programs live in the subconscious mind, playing in the background like a never-ending playlist you didn't choose. On the other hand, the conscious mind is where you can start taking the wheel, recognising those limitations, and rewriting the script. When we consciously shift how we think and respond, we open the door to new levels of awareness.

Your Higher Self

The term 'higher self' can be misleading because it is not higher than you; it is you. Think of your higher self as your inner guide, your compass. No, it's not a taller, shinier version of you! It's more like the wise mentor within you, always connected to your purpose and the deeper truths of your journey. Your higher self exists beyond your body, mind, and ego. This part of you sees the bigger picture, guiding you with clarity and love.

You might experience your higher self as a gut feeling, a wave of inspiration, or even a dream that leaves you with an undeniable sense of knowing. Sometimes, it whispers through synchronicities, or you notice those little coincidences that feel too perfect to ignore.

The beauty of connecting with your higher self is that it reminds you of who you truly are: infinite, wise, and full of potential. For many, it's hard to hear this inner voice amid the distractions and noise of daily life. But when you're in flow state, that connection becomes much clearer, as if you're standing on the bridge to the Field with nothing blocking the way.

The Field

We explored the Field in Chapter 1 as the infinite energy that connects everything. Some call it universal consciousness, source, or simply the All. Whatever name resonates with you, the Field is where all possibilities exist. The Field resonates as pure love, a frequency beyond space and time, where energy organises into coherence and creation begins. It's vast and deeply personal, holding the energy of creation and connection. The Field is an Infinite realm of energy and intelligence that holds more information than our everyday 3D reality. The Field offers us access to possibilities beyond what we perceive with our senses. Let's explore the science behind the Field's abundant information and discover how it far exceeds what our bodies can hold in the 3D world.

Scientists estimate that while the human brain can process up to 11 million bits of information per second, our conscious mind perceives only 40 to 50 bits — an almost negligible fraction of what's available (Zimmermann, 1986). This stark difference suggests our awareness barely scratches the surface, which aligns with the view of many researchers that physical reality itself is only a tiny fraction of what truly exists — our 3D world is like a single drop of water in an infinite ocean of intelligence, energy, and potential. Let me give you an analogy to help you understand how much information we can access in the Field.

Think about your smartphone. When connected to Wi-Fi, it can tap into a vast amount of information online. But if it's on flight mode or offline, your access is severely limited — you can only use what's already downloaded, like a few songs or books.

Now, imagine your phone is your body, and the internet is the Field. When you're stuck in limiting beliefs and old programming, your access to information is just as restricted. But when you shift your frequency and remove those blocks, you reconnect and tap into a limitless source of data — just like switching your phone back online. As we move into the next chapter, consider the abundance of information available when you tune into the Field to manifest your dreams.

I will reiterate a crucial point: We don't just experience or visit the Field — we are it. This is hard to get your head around, but once you grasp it, it is life-changing. We are information (waves of energy) in the Field that condenses into physical form (our body), much like how quantum particles exist as waves of possibility until observed. This means we are not physical beings generating consciousness, but we are consciousness that has taken form in our body. Our true essence exists first in the Field, and our bodies are simply a temporary, condensed expression of that energy. Just sit with that for a while. Look further into it if you need to; it helps you go deeper in meditation and helps you look at your life from a new perspective.

Always remember this: In a state of love, with an open heart and elevated emotions, you don't just connect to the Field — you will remember that you were never separate from it. This oneness is described by many as the feeling of coming home.

Other Layers?

Some describe additional layers such as the oversoul, soul clusters, or even higher dimensions than 5D, which I will describe next. While these are fascinating concepts, we won't delve into them in this book. If they intrigue you, plenty of material exists to explore further. For now, let's focus on what we can simplify and apply.

Levels of Awareness

When discussing different levels of awareness—often referred to as levels of consciousness—many people use terms like third, fourth or fifth dimensions (3D-5D) to describe how we experience life:

- **3D** is rooted in the material world, focused on survival and individuality. It's the realm of physicality, where we often feel separate and limited. In this dimension, everything operates within the constraints of time, space, and the speed of light. Therefore, 3D has a built-in ceiling — the speed of light acts as a limit. However, when reality shifts beyond this speed, we can access higher dimensions where energy, consciousness, and possibilities expand far beyond what we can perceive with our senses.

- **4D** is like a steppingstone between our old, limited perspectives in the 3D world and the unity of higher dimensions. It's the phase where we begin shifting our beliefs and dismantling limiting patterns. Time feels more fluid here, and our intuition grows stronger as we move beyond physical constraints, cultivating a more profound sense of awareness and presence.

- **5D** is the frequency of love, connection, and flow. Here, you begin to see the interconnectedness of everything and create from a place of unity and compassion. The focus shifts from separation to oneness, and reality becomes more fluid, responding effortlessly to your energy and intention. Time collapses, and the energy of instant manifestation is possible. You're shifting into a higher state of consciousness that transcends duality, fear, and ego-driven thinking. You're more attuned to The Field in this state because you operate from a space of love and unity rather than logic, separation, and conditioned patterns. You become less reactive to external chaos and more anchored in your internal state, making conscious creation easier. 5D level of awareness isn't just about being more connected to The Field — it's about realising that you ARE the Field, actively co-creating and influencing your reality in real-time.

These levels of awareness are not about 'levelling up' or escaping where you are. It's about expanding your perspective and experiencing life with more depth and connection. It's about remembering who you are. Our beliefs and trapped emotions can keep us rooted in the 3D world, making it harder to access higher dimensions. That's why working through the four steps in this book is so important. The steps help you release what holds you back, making the transition to a more expansive reality feel natural and effortless.

Remember, at the beginning of this chapter, we discussed that as a baby, we know we are oneness? So, to evolve spiritually, we must retrain ourselves to remember the truth we were born with: that we are inherently connected to everything. Our cells already know this, as biology operates in harmony with the interconnectedness of life. We must unlearn our conditioned mind and the ego's narrative of separation to return to this innate wisdom. When we align with this understanding, we reconnect with the wholeness of who we are.

You are more than your body and mind. You are a multidimensional being with infinite potential. The more you align with your higher self and the Field, the more you step into that potential. Speaking of our multidimensional nature, consider this:

What if our journey towards *Opposite World* reshapes not just now but also our future and past selves? What if the new frequencies we are creating ripple across all our timelines? While our 3D experience appears linear, quantum science hints at retrocausality (the possibility that the future can influence the past.) I won't dive into this concept too deeply here because it's quite a stretch. However, I will say this: while writing this book, I had an aha!

moment. Actually, I had many. One of the most striking realisations was about those unexpected sparks of joy I felt in moments when I should have been in despair. Looking back, I wonder……. *was that my future self sending a whisper of hope?* I believe so; I feel my work now affects all my timelines. I also think I went through tough times to give me the wisdom to write this book, which, in turn, will help others.

This is a vast topic, far too expansive for this book alone; the mystery beckons me to keep exploring, stay tuned!

We still haven't explained a couple of key terms: your soul and consciousness. How do these all fit together? I'll give you a visual.

Imagine your soul as a glowing orb — pure energy in its natural state. The soul takes on a more tangible, particle-like form in your body. Now, picture your higher self as the radiant light shining from the orb, illuminating your path and offering guidance. Finally, there's consciousness — your awareness. It acts as the bridge, accessing information from the Field and enabling you to navigate and interact with the world. In essence, the soul provides the foundation, the higher self offers direction, and consciousness is the mechanism that ties it all together.

Understanding these layers lets you see how they all work together to unlock creativity and transformation. You'll also find this knowledge handy when we explore meditation and manifestation in upcoming chapters. Remember, these layers aren't separate boxes but different expressions of the same infinite essence. I will declare that this is how I see our layers; you may see it differently. So, take what resonates, leave what doesn't, and remember that your growth and transformation are uniquely yours. And always, always choose love. It's the clearest path to connection, creation, and flow. Before we end this chapter, let's take it a little further and step outside the life we are in now and ponder if there will be more.

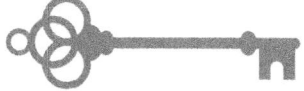

We are the universe observing itself through our eyes.

Is This Your Only Life?

Since we've touched on the idea of the soul, I can't resist diving into the fascinating yet sometimes controversial topic of reincarnation. It's not a mainstream topic, but this is *Opposite World*, so we're going there. Everyone has their take on this subject, often shaped by personal experiences, cultural or religious beliefs, societal programming, or maybe it's something you've never given much thought to. For me, I believe this isn't our only life. My belief was solidified after an extraordinary experience when my firstborn daughter's soul visited me before she was even conceived. It was a profound, life-altering moment; to this day, I know it was undeniably real.

Many cultures have long believed that our lives are connected across multiple lifetimes, like threads in a bigger picture. I'm sure you can find thousands of stories online of people who say they can remember their past lives. I want to bring some science to you on this subject. For over 60 years, the University of Virginia's Division of Perceptual Studies (DOPS) has conducted groundbreaking research investigating many mysteries of human consciousness. As well as reincarnation, DOPS also explores phenomena such as near-death experiences, altered states of consciousness, and the neuroscience of psychic abilities — all of these challenge mainstream scientific paradigms.

To give a brief on their reincarnation studies, they have studied cases of around 2,500 young children aged two to six years who recall details of past lives. The children studied remember precise information about a previous life, such as names, locations, and events. Many of these details have been verified as accurate despite the children having no apparent way of knowing the information. You can go through the university's website to see their work; the link is at the end of the book. I will give you one example of a case discussed by a child psychiatrist at the University, Dr Jim B Tucker; he has details in his book. The child studied is James Leininger, a young boy from Louisiana. He began having vivid nightmares about plane crashes at the age of two. He provided detailed accounts of being a World War II pilot named James (interestingly, same name) who flew a Corsair aircraft that was shot down over Iwo Jima. James also mentioned specific details, such as the name of a fellow pilot, 'Jack Larsen,' and the ship they operated from, the 'Natoma.' His parents were initially sceptical but then researched these claims and discovered that a World War II aircraft carrier, the USS Natoma Bay, had participated in the Battle of Iwo Jima. They also found records of a pilot named James Huston Jr., who indeed was killed in action during that battle.

Additionally, it checked out that a pilot named Jack Larsen served alongside Huston. This was one of many cases that intrigues the researchers at DOPS. That story blows my mind!

What if life is more expansive than we've been taught? Could exploring these possibilities unlock new layers of who we truly are? Could new beliefs help us live more relaxed, joyful lives? I admire universities that support their experts in exploring research beyond the mainstream and blending science with spirituality. I hope more courageous individuals continue to step forward and challenge the boundaries of conventional thought in all areas.

When reincarnation is described, it often centres around the idea that our essence or consciousness transcends the boundaries of a single lifetime. As explained throughout this book, our consciousness isn't just contained within us — it's interconnected with everything. There are many examples suggesting this might be the case. For instance, organ transplant recipients' reports describe experiencing their donors' memories, preferences, or even personality traits. This phenomenon, often called 'cellular memory,' raises fascinating questions about how information and consciousness might extend beyond the brain and the body. This concept ties in beautifully with the idea of water memory that we discussed in Chapter 4, where water is believed to retain information beyond its physical properties. Just as water may hold the essence of what it encounters, perhaps our consciousness operates similarly, connecting us to a greater web of existence. Oneness is the key!

If you want to explore reincarnation further, I recommend Dr. Michael Newton's Journey of the Souls. Newton shares insights into the afterlife through the accounts of clients he guided into deep hypnosis. Using regression therapy, Newton explores what happens to souls between lives, revealing detailed descriptions of the spiritual realm, the process of soul development, and the experiences souls have as they prepare for their next incarnation. It's an interesting read, and many people's stories are very similar.

Stay with me if that topic feels outside your comfort zone because it could offer you peace. If research suggests that we're here to learn lessons and heal wounds, maybe that information could shift our perspective. If the fear of death is holding us down in lower emotions, perhaps knowing that we don't die, our bodies do, could lighten the load. If our soul is energy, it can't be destroyed; it merely changes form. This is because it can express itself as energy in the Field or as particles in a new body. Instead of saying, 'We only have one life,' what if we don't? What if our work today helps us now and prepares us for whatever comes next? Some believe that fully healing in this life means we graduate from Earth school. Others suggest that our soul aims to clear up the wounds to live in a higher state of consciousness.

Whether or not you believe in past or future lives, there's no harm in being curious. In *Opposite World*, we always leave the door open to possibilities because, in the end, none of us hold the ultimate truth. So, why lock ourselves into rigid beliefs? Growth comes from expansion, not contraction. Throughout this book, I'm sharing my personal description of our reality, not a prescription for yours. It's a description, not a prescription. I'm a forever student, learning something new every day, and I encourage you to be the same. Beliefs should evolve as we do. Seek your own understanding, challenge your perspectives, and allow yourself the freedom to explore — because staying curious is the only belief worth holding onto.

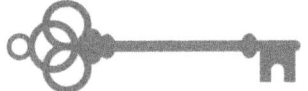

We are infinite consciousness having
a human experience.

CHAPTER 8

LIFE BY DESIGN

(Spoiler alert: The Secret left out some secrets regarding the Law of Attraction.)

Creating Your Dream Life

Let's step into the dessert section of this journey — where we create dreams. Have you ever tried to manifest something like your dream job, a perfect relationship, or financial abundance, only to feel like the universe wasn't picking up your order? It's time to figure out why. Before we break it down, let's look at Kate's story.

Kate had been dreaming of finding her new partner. She tried everything: made a list of what she was looking for, crafted vision boards, full moon rituals, burnt pieces of her hair (I think I made that one up — she didn't do that, sorry, Kate). Despite all her efforts, every time she went on a date, it seemed like they had escaped the crazy farm. After each date, she couldn't help but vent to her friends, saying things like, 'I only ever attract people who are completely off their rocker!' Without realising it, her words were programming her reality. Her world mirrored her deepest thoughts and beliefs, not her neatly written list of dream-partner qualities. You see, the creative energy around us doesn't distinguish between fact and fiction. It simply amplifies what you're consistently thinking, saying, and feeling. Kate was putting out the wrong energy, and her list was holding her back. Her list also called in what she didn't want; she had written: '*I don't want any more crazy guys! He can't be emotionally unstable.*' All the Field could hear was crazy and unstable. I think you get the point where Kate was going wrong. Kate's story reminds you to check in with the narratives you're creating. Are your thoughts aligned with what you truly want, or are they accidentally reinforcing what you don't want?

If, like Kate, you are disheartened by your manifestations, you are not alone. Many people approach manifestation with great hope, only to be left disillusioned when their desires remain out of reach or appear for a moment and then disappear. The truth is that manifestation is oversimplified. It's not just about wishful thinking or positive vibes. It's about alignment; we need all the ducks to line up to be successful. We learnt about your values, thoughts, and emotions and how the collectiveness of all of these creates energy or the frequency at which you vibrate. Many teachings skip the crucial groundwork, leaving people feeling unworthy or not good at it.

Remember the documentary *The Secret*? Its popularity soared, introducing millions to the law of attraction. I still remember in the early 2000s when my neighbour left a CD of *The Secret* on my doorstep, like some mystical message meant just for me. Watching it, I felt an instant connection. It validated something I'd always believed but had never managed to put into words.

While *The Secret* was undoubtedly inspiring, manifesting goes beyond positive thinking and visualisation. It delves deeper into the essence of who you are. To truly manifest your desires, you must embody the emotions of what you want as if it's already happening. Just as we learnt about feeling the energy of a negative emotion to dissolve it, the same principle applies when manifesting. Emotions are energy and act as a bridge to your desires in the Field. Paired with your thoughts, which carry the information, this energy creates a powerful connection to what you seek. Misalignment can create roadblocks, whether stemming from trapped emotions or a disconnect from your values. This is why chapters 3 to 6 were crucial to understand before we delve into this chapter. If you have resistance in your subconscious, your wish will not be granted. Or it may be granted for a moment but then taken away from you because you haven't held it in the right frequency.

Years ago, I learnt this hard lesson. I manifested a certain amount of money I had written on a vision board. In a very short time, I achieved the exact dollar value in equity on properties. I never managed to hold it because one aspect of my life was out of balance. Remember doing the Alignment Life Tracker in Chapter 3? I had an area that had a gaping hole. I also had not learnt some lessons and was using the success of money as a shield to protect myself from hidden emotions.

The Science Backing Manifestation

Another point is that manifesting isn't like the genie in the bottle, where you only get one wish. The good news is that endless possibilities await you in the Field. So, there isn't just one tiramisu waiting for you; it's a buffet of desserts. I'll get a bit 'sciencey' again for those who need it.

Don't just sit back and assume life will unfold on autopilot; you have more control than that. Quantum physics shows us that we live in a universe of probabilities, not fixed destinies — you have more control than you think. According to the multiverse theory, multiple realities exist simultaneously, each shaped by different choices and states of consciousness. As we dive into the science of manifesting, let's revisit the observer effect, which we touched on in Chapter 1. In quantum mechanics, this phenomenon demonstrates that the act of observation influences the behaviour of particles. Some interpret this as evidence that consciousness has the power to shape reality. Moreover, neuroscience shows that our brain's reticular activating system (RAS) filters information based on our focus. When you repeatedly think about a goal and pair it with the emotions of already achieving it, your RAS notices opportunities that align with your desires. Essentially, you are programming your mind to work harmoniously with your environment to bring your vision to life (Pfaff et al., 2008).

～

This isn't magic — it's a synergy of intention, emotion, and aligned action. So, if multiple realities exist, we have a series of potential outcomes waiting for us in the Field. You must agree this is very exciting! Each potential is accessible through the choices we make and the emotions we embody. When we align our energy, we resonate with a specific timeline that considers those possibilities. So, what is it that you want? Do you feel worthy of it? Can you imagine it? Can you feel it? Are you taking action towards it? If so, then your wish will be granted!

Creating Abundance

Abundance is one of the most common things people try to manifest. For many, this means financial wealth; really, though, you can be abundant in anything. At its heart, the desire for abundance is often about achieving freedom. To manifest it, you must create energy that aligns with abundance, feel the emotions of already having it, and clear any hidden blocks that might stand in your way.

Remember the section of this book on your money mindset? It won't work if you have negative thoughts about people who have money and abundance. You also need to dissolve any unworthy emotions. Remember that you can not create abundance from lack. Another step is to go out and start taking action to get that abundance. Be open to all opportunities that pop up because you never know how your manifestations will show up. Abundant people are self-starters and aren't afraid to take risks or fail. They jump in.

Take note: there is a caveat to manifesting money or abundance. While many believe the key lies in overcoming feelings of unworthiness and feeling the emotion of already having it, there's another important principle at play: the law of reciprocity. This law reminds us that to manifest abundance, we must allow ourselves to receive with gratitude and ease. If discomfort arises when receiving, it disrupts the balance, creating resistance and blocking the flow of abundance into your life.

So, the next time you receive something, whether it's a compliment, a gift, or financial support, embrace it. Be okay with receiving, welcome it fully, and remind yourself that you are deserving. By doing so, you honour the flow of giving and receiving, allowing abundance to flourish.

~

Let us list the steps for manifesting anything you want. You cannot miss any of these steps.

Key Steps of Manifestation

1. **Write it Down:** Define your desires and goals. Be specific. This step is essential; your angels above do not know what you want unless you are clear about it. If you keep it in your head, it gets all jumbled. Please write it down! Then, read it out loud and in your head. Walk around with your notes and read them often. You must write down what you want as if you already have it and express your gratitude. For example: *Dear God, I am so grateful for my new fantastic job, which pays me double what I used to earn, offers me the balanced lifestyle I require and matches all my values.* You can give much more detail than that.

2. **Feel the Emotion:** Connect deeply with the feeling of already having what you desire. Connect it to your heart and feel joy whenever you think about it.

3. **Visualise:** Get creative. Picture yourself with what you desire, play a movie in your head or make one on your computer if that's your thing. Use as much detail as you can. As you walk down the street, visualise that you already have it

and how you would walk and feel. You could even create a vision board if that helps.

4. **Align Your Energy:** Match your thoughts, emotions, and actions with the frequency of your vision. If you are trying to manifest abundance, don't walk around in lack.

5. **Check Your Values:** Ensure your goals align with your core values.

6. **Believe You are Worthy:** Cultivate a deep sense of deservingness.

7. **Create Away from Distractions when Possible:** Sit with your dreams during quiet moments, such as in flow state, prayer or meditation. Manifestation happens faster when you're present, not lost in the noise of everyday life.

8. **Take Inspired Action:** Take purposeful steps toward your vision. You can't just wait for it to arrive; you must do something. For example, if you want to buy a car, open a bank account and start saving. Then, look at cars online in the price category you want.

Use all your senses to embed your dreams so that you activate all parts of your brain. You don't have to worry about how you will get something; that's not your job. If you do all the above steps, the Field will surprise you.

DREAM Your Reality

To remember these steps, use the acronym DREAM:

- **D** - Define your desires.

- **R** - Resonate with the emotions of having them.

- **E** - Energise your alignment.

- **A** - Align with your values.

- **M** - Move toward it with inspired action.

When Is the Best Time to Create Your Dream Life?

The short answer? Anytime and all the time. Manifestation isn't something you schedule like a dentist appointment. It's something you weave into your life. Whether you're enjoying a quiet moment, grocery shopping, drifting off to sleep, or deep in meditation (we'll talk more about that in the next chapter), the key is to carry the energy of your dreams with you wherever you go. Keep a notepad beside your bed because as you meditate and spend more time in the Field, you may get messages in your dreams. Trust me, you won't remember them, so write them down. They could be the keys to the dreams you are creating.

Here's the key: Walk like your dreams are already your reality. Speak as though you've already achieved them. Skip the 'one day, I will...' and go straight to 'I am...' Feel the emotions of your future.

The new you is walking down the street, grinning like you just won the lottery, feeling excited because you know your vision is coming. People might look at you and think you've got a secret because you do. You're living in alignment with your dreams, clearing your bridge to the Field, and that's where the magic happens. You're living in *Opposite World*, where dreams come true. All you need is a vibrational match to what you want to create.

Mars, Venus and Intention Setting

This concept is something I have thought about for a while, and I started paying attention to the people around me. Do you remember the book *Men Are from Mars, Women Are from Venus*? It highlighted how men and women often communicate differently. These differences go beyond the verbal and extend to our energetic communication. Women tend to excel at multitasking, weaving together complex, interconnected thoughts. They do better in this state than concentrating on one thing. While men often thrive with singular, laser-focused concentration. Of course, I am generalising here, and we are all unique, but it's a thought to consider when setting intentions in the Field. Perhaps women could benefit from envisioning a full, vibrant scenario with all its details, while men might achieve better results by focusing on one key object or outcome. Embracing these natural strengths could enhance your ability to align with and manifest your desires effectively.

Avoiding the Pitfalls of Manifestation

Manifestation isn't just about dreaming big and watching magic happen; it requires balance, awareness, and a strong foundation. Along the way, a few common pitfalls can throw things off course. We have mentioned some 'what not to do' strategies, but here are more. Let's talk about them.

- **Align Values** - First, ensure your goals align with your core values (remember, we have done this exercise and know our highest values). Imagine manifesting a high-powered job that sounds amazing on paper but clashes with your deep desire for family time and freedom. Even if you succeed, you might find that the outcome doesn't bring the hoped-for happiness. Always ask yourself, 'Does this align with what matters most to me'? When your goals and values are in harmony, everything flows more naturally.

- **Forget the How** - Another big trap is getting hung up on how your manifestation will happen. Controlling every step can lead to frustration and limit the Field's ability to surprise you! Remember, your job is to define what you want and take inspired action, and it will unfold in its own way. Trust the process and leave some room for magic. You don't need to know how you will get something. You just have to put your order in. If your dream is a big one, you could break it into steps. For instance, if you want $1,000,000, you could say, In 3 months, I will have $300,000, etc. You are creating a timeline to get there, but you don't need to know the 'how.'

- **Have Patience** - Let's be honest. We've all wanted instant results at some point. But manifestation is like planting a seed; it may need time to grow. If you dig it up every five minutes to see if it's sprouting, you'll only slow things down. Stay patient and trust the timing.

- **Feel Worthy** - One of the sneakiest pitfalls is self-doubt or feeling unworthy. If deep down you believe you don't deserve what you're manifesting, that energy can block it from coming into your life. Manifestation thrives on confidence and self-worth, so it's worth doing the inner work to believe you truly deserve your goals.

- **Balance is the Key** - It's not enough to manifest something; you need a stable base to sustain it. If your life is out of balance or you carry unresolved emotions, it's like building a house on shaky ground. Take time to align your inner and outer worlds. It makes all the difference in holding onto what you create.

- **Don't Yearn** -Yearning for something can unintentionally create an energy of lack, signalling to the Field that you don't already have what you desire. Desperation blocks the flow of manifestation because it focuses your energy on what's missing rather than what's possible. Instead of yearning, focus on gratitude and contentment for what you already have. This doesn't mean giving up on your dreams; it means aligning with them from a place of abundance. Manifestation works best when you embody the emotions of already having what you desire, allowing it to flow naturally to you. Think of it as attracting, not chasing.

The same principle applies when in the dating world. Avoid sending out desperate energy by yearning for or clinging to the idea of love. Instead, vibrate in love and abundance, and you'll naturally attract energy that matches your own.

Remember, manifestation is about co-creation. When you align your energy, values, and actions, you're not just calling in your dreams but building a life that can hold them. You will then naturally open yourself to receive when you enter this state of being.

Plot Twist

Here's something to consider: What if the things you manifest aren't aligned with your highest good? Or what if the universe has something far better waiting for you in the Field?

Manifestation isn't about clinging to one specific outcome; it's about stepping into flow and letting life unfold like an exciting movie. Focusing too narrowly on one outcome might block a better possibility or miss the signs guiding you toward what truly aligns. Here's a surface example: imagine you're manifesting that top-of-the-line Toyota. You've visualised it, felt the emotions, and worked toward it. But in another timeline, you're cruising in a Porsche. By focusing only on the Toyota, you might block that possibility. So dream high, my friend!

The takeaway? DREAM, feel, and act, but leave space for the Field to surprise you. Let the Field meet you halfway. Sometimes, what's in store is far better than anything imaginable.

'As a man thinketh in his heart, so is he.' — Proverbs 23:7

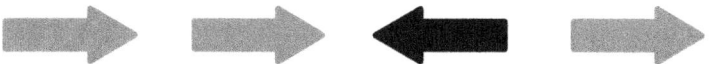

CHAPTER 9

MEDITATION

Here it is, the topic you've either been eagerly awaiting or quietly dreading. Meditation is a fun and exciting tool for transformation. Have you tried it, or is it something you've been avoiding with excuses like:

'I don't have time to meditate'

'I can't sit with my thoughts'

'I can't sit still'

'I've tried it, it's just not for me'?

If you've said anything similar, I have news for you! You're exactly the person who should meditate.

The Benefits of Meditation

Before we dive into the details, let's look at what meditation offers you. What are the benefits of meditation? There are so many, and it's impossible to list them all. The benefits differ for everyone, and it's essential to understand that **meditation will offer you what you need.** You'll get a sense of this when you read the stories of regular meditators later in this chapter. But here's a taste of what meditation can do:

- Regulates your nervous system
- Ignite your intuition
- Helps you sleep better
- Reverses aging (seriously, it's anti-aging magic)
- Connects you to your higher self and the Field
- Keeps you in flow state after meditating
- Your dreams become more vivid or even lucid
- Compassion and kindness increase
- Heals trauma and disease
- Calms anger and reduces anxiety
- Helps beat addictions
- Boost optimism and joy
- Tunes you into higher frequencies
- Attunes you to inner guidance and wisdom
- Create a sense of oneness and peace
- Helps you escape your overthinking brain
- Brings you closer to your soul's purpose
- Allows you to have supernatural experiences
- Allows you to see life through the eyes of the Field
- Create alpha-dominant brain waves instead of beta
- Enhanced learning and memory

- Calms your blood pressure, respiratory rate, and heart rate
- Get beyond the analytical thinking mind
- Unlocks the door to the quantum world
- Expands awareness beyond the physical, accessing more profound states of consciousness and higher dimensions
- Your heart will become open and coherent

Okay, I could keep going, but you get the idea that meditation is a powerhouse.

Once you get over the initial awkwardness and stick with it, meditation becomes an active and transformative experience. It's the one distraction that's genuinely good for your body, mind, and spirit. Meditation allows you to become a vessel for something greater, a higher level of consciousness that is love. When you allow this connection, prepare for it to change your life.

The deeper you go with your meditations, the more you change — your perception of life shifts. You begin to tap into intuition and inner knowing that's always been there but now feels fully alive. Conversations deepen. You stop just hearing people's words and start feeling the truth behind them, sensing their essence. You see through people's words, actions, and struggles with newfound compassion, and suddenly, the world looks much more loving. Your nervous system calms down, and you notice the background noise disappearing. You start to see the world through the eyes of the Field, birthing consciousness through your body. You will become limitless.

Think about the work we have been doing with letting go of emotions and changing our thought patterns and beliefs; it can be hard work, right? If you can learn to connect to the Field in meditation, you can do this work much quicker because you are working with energy, no matter what. I have witnessed many people moving stuck emotions in their bodies through meditation. When I first witnessed this, I found it quite disturbing, but after learning about it and speaking to people who experience it, I've realised it's profound and is like the ultimate biohack.

You often get surprising nudges and synchronicities when you are in sync with the Field. The more you meditate, the more you align with the Field and get to know yourself — your true self, on a level you may never have imagined possible.

What Science Says About Meditation

The fact is that people who practice meditation report improvements in their overall well-being. This isn't just perception; studies by many scientists show that you can physically see changes in the brain using brain imaging technology, like electroencephalography (EEG), when people are or have been meditating. A documentary that came out in 2024 called *The Source: It's Within You* shows evidence of the extensive physical and mental changes to meditators. The studies were and are still being conducted by scientists from two universities in the USA who follow the same protocols as pharmaceutical studies. I highly recommend you watch this, especially if you are new to meditation and the Field.

As we have discovered in previous chapters, science suggests that memory storage may not be confined solely to neurons in the brain. This shows we can access information beyond the brain and from the Field. If true, meditation provides a unique opportunity to tap into this vast reservoir of information, allowing us to reprogram and realign our minds and bodies from a space beyond our usual mental constructs. As mentioned, the Field holds vast information beyond what our five senses can perceive in the 3D world. Studies in quantum mechanics and consciousness research suggest that meditation enhances access to this information by shifting brainwave states, increasing coherence, and allowing deeper intuitive insights.

So, we can access information in the Field; what else can we do? There are so many things, but here's an interesting fact. We can only see and hear a tiny amount of what exists in the world; in fact, it is a mere 0.0000001016%. Really think about that for a moment; it's crazy to get your head around! It emphasises how incredibly small our sensory perception range is compared to the vastness of what's out there. I think that is exciting. I'll break down that small percentage for you. The visible light range is just 430–770 THz, accounting for just 0.00034% of the electromagnetic spectrum. Similarly, the sounds we can hear are just 20–20,000 Hz, representing a mere 0.0000002% of the broader sound frequency spectrum.

These crazy low percentages mean an overwhelming amount of activity and energy is outside our sensory awareness. By quieting the mind and focusing inward during meditation, we can heighten our sensitivity and become attuned to subtle phenomena beyond these sensory limits. How is it possible we can tap into these senses? There are many reasons, but here are just three explanations:

- The brain's natural adaptability (neuroplasticity), which allows it to rewire and enhance sensory perception
- The subconscious mind processes vast amounts of information beyond our conscious awareness

- The synchronisation of the heart and brain may amplify our sensitivity to energy and frequencies around us.

These may explain why people often experience unexplainable sensations or insights in meditative states. I draw this science to your attention for two reasons:

1. So you can believe you can do much more than your current programming in the 3D world;
2. So you can understand the experiences our meditators have in the upcoming stories.

How to Meditate

The beauty of meditation is that there's not one right way to do it. You can explore many styles and teachings, but keep it simple to start with. The most important thing is to get started, even if it's just for a few minutes. Sometimes, you feel like you didn't 'achieve' anything, but remember, it will always be worth it.

Some people sit quietly, others lie down, and some even meditate while walking (yes, they keep their eyes open). You might listen to guided meditations, calming music, or specific frequencies. The main goal is to get out of your busy mind, tune in to the Field, elevate your emotions and let your outer world dissolve. Some people take months or years to get out of their busy heads; this is normal.

I find Dr. Joe Dispenza's meditations and the theories behind them profoundly transformative. Other excellent methods I recommend include The Silva Method by José Silva, Bob Proctor's teachings, Jerry Sergeant's Star Magic, Vipassana by Mr. Goenka, and the work of Deepak Chopra — the list goes on. You can even find excellent resources for meditation on some apps on your phone. Just a word of caution: steer clear of any AI-generated copies of well-known teachers. They might be using the wrong frequencies, and let's face it, no one wants their meditation session derailed by a glitchy algorithm!

There are so many different styles of meditation that it may take a while to find the one that best suits you. I recommend exploring a mix of techniques to experience different approaches. If you're new, start simple: focus on being still and letting go of your thinking mind.

If you're more experienced, here are some methods you could try.

Energy Alignment Methods
Working Through Your Chakras

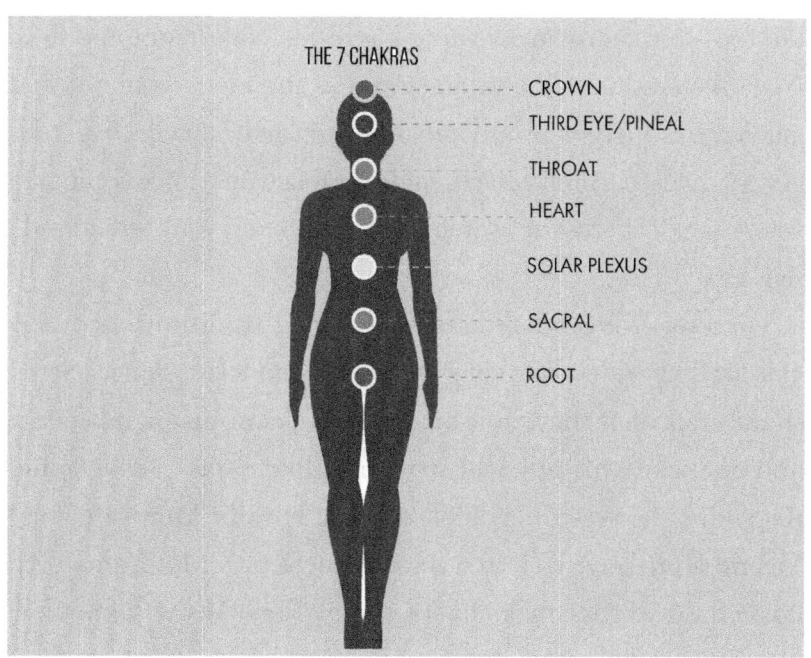

You've probably heard of chakras, often described as energy centres within the body that play a key role in our emotional, physical, and spiritual balance. See the image to see where they are located. I won't go too heavily into these little gifts within us; a lot is involved, but let's keep it simple. Focusing on them during meditation can help release stuck emotions, restore harmony, and bring a sense of coherence to both the mind and body. We discussed methods of having a coherent heart. You can use the same method to work on other energy centres. Remember when we discussed how information is stored in cells throughout your body, and we used tools to dissolve trapped emotions? Meditating through the chakras offers another powerful way to release and realign, helping you tap into your natural energy flow.

How do you work on these chakras in meditation? Remember, where focus goes, energy flows, so focus on where you feel the need. You might visualise each chakra and guide energy from the root to the crown, creating a sense of alignment and flow. Negative emotions are often stored in the lower chakras, and guiding this energy upward and outward can be an effective strategy for release. Alternatively, you can focus on a specific chakra where you feel tension or imbalance, directing your attention to that area.

Chakras, long recognised in Eastern traditions, are now gaining attention and being studied in modern science. Some studies hint that they emit measurable electromagnetic energy and connect with physical structures like nerve plexuses and the endocrine system. Trailblazers like Hiroshi Motoyama and Valerie Hunt have explored these mysteries — Motoyama even created devices to track chakra energy flow. At the same time,

Hunt linked emotional states and energy fields to the activity of the chakra system. More recent research suggests chakras might not just be metaphors but are detectable parts of our energetic makeup, tying into modern ideas like biofield therapy and energy medicine (Matos et al., 2021). These findings suggest that what was once considered purely spiritual may also have a foundation in bioelectromagnetics and cellular regulation. Can you see the threads weaving together ancient wisdom and modern science? Perhaps the answers we seek have always been within reach, waiting for us to rediscover and understand them through a new lens.

We discussed types of emotions in Chapter 4 and how negative emotions can be trapped in your body. For instance, you may have fear stuck in the root chakra, not speaking your truth in the throat chakra or grief in the heart chakra. Working with these energy centres can be an excellent tool for releasing these emotions or helping those areas become more coherent. How do you do that? In brief, without doing a whole day course with you, you can guide healing and balance by focusing on these energy centres during meditation. I'll repeat this: Where your focus goes, energy flows. Concentrating on a particular chakra is observing it and actively nurturing and energising it.

Whether guided or not, working on your chakras during meditation is a great way to create coherence throughout your body, release emotions, and allow you to focus on something away from your thinking mind. When I work on balancing my energy centres in meditation, I sometimes feel jolts of energy. This is especially noticeable when creating coherence amongst them all at once.

Sound Frequencies

Sound has long been a bridge between the physical and the spiritual, offering unique pathways to meditation through rhythm, frequency, and resonance. Among these, binaural beats, isochronic tones, and solfeggio frequencies stand out as powerful tools for enhancing focus, relaxation, and connection to the deeper self.

Binaural Beats rely on two slightly different frequencies played separately in each ear to create brainwave entrainment. For this, you'll need headphones. Interestingly, binaural beats were explored in the CIA's Gateway Program — a training system developed by the Monroe Institute to alter consciousness and expand states of awareness. One of the areas of interest the CIA was developing with this program was remote viewing (CIA, 1983). What's that? It's the ability to take your consciousness (awareness) to other locations. To expand, it is the practice of using focused consciousness to perceive or gather information about a distant or unseen target beyond normal sensory perception. The CIA used this method to spy or assess the safety of areas without physically being there. While this fascinating concept is outside the scope of this book, it's something to ponder when considering just how powerful we can truly be.

Isochronic Tones use rhythmic pulses of sound at specific frequencies. Different frequencies of isochronic tones are associated with various brainwave states. For example, tracks pulsing at 7.83 Hz match the Earth's natural frequency, also known as the Schumann resonance, which many people find particularly grounding. Listening to this frequency in meditation fosters a calm, harmonious state, aligning the listener with the Earth's resonance.

Solfeggio Frequencies rooted in ancient traditions, are a set of specific sound frequencies believed to influence the mind and body. The term *Solfeggio* comes from a musical system used for vocal training, and these tones are often linked to Gregorian chants —sacred hymns sung by monks in medieval Christianity. These frequencies are thought to interact with the body's energy centres (chakras) to promote balance and well-being, with each frequency carrying unique healing properties that may affect physical, mental, and emotional states. Here are some examples:

396 Hz: Releases guilt and fear.

417 Hz: Encourages change and clears negative energy.

528 Hz: Known as the 'miracle tone,' associated with DNA repair and transformation.

639 Hz: Strengthens relationships and fosters connection and love.

741 Hz: Detoxifies the body and mind.

852 Hz: Enhances intuition and awakens inner strength.

963 Hz: Connects to higher consciousness or the divine.

Another chant I love and beautifully illustrates the spiritual connection to sound is the Lotus Sutra (Buddhist). This chant has deeply meditative and transformational properties. It represents purity and spiritual awakening, symbolising the lotus flower rising from the mud. Nikko Hansen has created a stunning rendition of this chant, which you can find on YouTube. It blends ancient tradition with modern sound healing techniques. Listening to it can evoke peace, clarity, and connection to the Field.

All these sounds can help calm the mind, harmonise the body, and ease you into a meditative state.

Heart and Brain Coherence

This technique involves syncing the heart and brain to create harmony and balance. We do this by focusing on these areas and feeling elevated emotions like gratitude or love while breathing slowly and deeply. This can align these two powerful centres and allow you to access more profound clarity and calm. We have already learnt about heart coherence in Chapter 2. Focusing on this in your morning meditations can help create a beautiful state for the whole day.

Matching the Frequency of Your Manifestations

We've just wrapped up a chapter on creating your dream life through manifestation, but there's an important point I want to highlight. When you are in *the Field*, time as we know it doesn't exist. This means that if you connect with the frequency of your dreams while meditating, those dreams can manifest very quickly in your outer world. In the 3D world, thoughts and feelings can take much longer to ripple back to you. This delay can be a blessing, especially when starting with thought sculpting and manifesting. It gives you more time to refine, adjust, and play with the energy of your desires. However, these time lapses in the physical world can also create illusions. People often don't realise that something they manifested has arrived because so much time has passed since they initially set the intention. They might call it luck or coincidence, never realising their own thought patterns created it.

Meditation offers a unique advantage because it allows you to bypass time constraints. In the Field, things can unfold faster, and you become more aware of your role as the creator of your reality. I've heard many people say they just knew when they connected to the frequency of their manifestations during meditation. It's a feeling of certainty that resonates deeply, almost like hitting the perfect note in a song. I do this all the time … I'm referring to the perfect singing, although my family would disagree. Think of the connection you feel when drawing in your manifestation as tuning in to a radio station. The clearer your signal — your intention and emotion — the stronger the connection. The Field doesn't work with 'someday' or 'maybe.' It responds to the energy you're emitting right now. When you radiate the emotions of already living your dream life, you collapse the time it takes for that vision to materialise in the 3D world.

Are you curious about how this works in real life? Our meditators, who bring this concept to life, will soon share some incredible manifestation stories.

Everyone has their style and what works for them when meditating; there is no right or wrong. However, I have put together some tips that may help you.

Meditation Tips

1. **Wear a Mask** No, not the superhero kind (unless that's your thing). A simple eye mask can help block distractions and keep your focus inward.

2. **Minimise Distractions** Make sure your space is as distraction-free as possible —keep phones on silent, pets entertained, and doors closed. Tell anyone in your house that you are meditating and ask them not to disturb you.

3. **Handle Intrusive Thoughts** When thoughts pop up (and trust me, they will), don't fight them. Simply notice them and let them go. Picture yourself gently pushing them down and off to the side, or use a word like 'cancel' to dissolve them. It might feel impossible at first, but your focus will improve over time with practice.

4. **Focus on Your Breath** If you ever feel overwhelmed, just return to your breath. Let everything else go for now — breathing alone can be a powerful meditation.

5. **Get Comfortable** Make sure you're seated (or lying down) comfortably and that the temperature of your space feels just right. I like to sit on a comfortable chair. Leave the lying down meditations for when you are more experienced; otherwise, you might fall asleep.

6. **Take a Pre-Meditation Bathroom Break** Trust me; nothing interrupts deep meditation like realising you need the toilet halfway through.

7. **Have a Game Plan** Decide what you'll focus on before you start, whether it will be manifesting, healing, or just connecting with the Field. Having a plan before you start can stop your brain from wandering. Do all the thinking outside of meditation so the left brain can rest.

8. **Set a Timer** If you are not doing a guided meditation and you're worried about losing track of time or checking the

clock, set a gentle timer. This way, you can relax fully without wondering how long you've been meditating.

9. **Use a Comfortable Cushion or Chair** If you're sitting, invest in a meditation cushion or chair that supports good posture while keeping you comfortable. A numb leg can pull you right out of your Zen!

10. **Meditate in Nature** If you can access a quiet spot outdoors, try meditating in nature. The sounds of birds, rustling leaves, or flowing water can deepen your connection. Having beautiful natural sounds also allows you to put your focus on them, taking your mind out of your body.

11. **Don't Judge Your Experience** Some meditations feel amazing, while others feel like a wrestling match with your mind. Both are valid, and both are part of the process. You will come up against yourself; honour that, and don't judge it; awareness is everything. Keep reminding yourself that no meditation you do is ever bad — that is just your judgment. Every meditation you do is worth it, and something is changing in you, whether you can see it or not.

12. **Celebrate Small Wins** Whether you managed to sit still for the first time or you are feeling slightly calmer in your outer world, acknowledge and celebrate your progress. Meditation is a journey, not a competition.

13. **Smile While You Meditate** Even if you don't feel all that happy, try smiling during meditation. It can help lift your energy closer to the frequency of love, making it easier to connect with the Field.

14. **Incorporate Music or Frequencies** If you are not doing a guided meditation, play some soft music or frequencies. These can help create a calming atmosphere and enhance your experience.

15. **Shift Your Gaze Upward** With your eyes closed, gently angle your eyeballs upward about 20 degrees. This subtle movement can help guide you into Alpha brain waves, a state perfect for meditation and relaxation. It's like giving your brain a nudge towards calm focus.

16. **Learn Breathing Techniques** Experiment with breathing techniques like box breathing (inhale for four counts, hold for four counts, exhale for four counts, and hold for four counts). These methods can calm your nervous system, sharpen your focus, and make it easier to settle into meditation.

17. **Clear Your To-Do List** If there's a nagging task on your mind, like answering that email or putting the clothes in the dryer — take care of it before you meditate. Clearing these minor distractions beforehand helps you fully relax and focus without mental interruptions.

18. **Start with an Elevated Emotion** Begin your meditation by focusing on elevated emotions like love or gratitude. If it's hard to access those feelings, think of a person, pet or memory that fills you with joy. If you notice your energy dropping to lower frequencies during meditation, gently bring that image or thought back to raise your vibration again. Don't forget your heart coherence.

The Power of Group Meditations

Group meditations are incredibly potent. The idea is simple: when large groups meditate together, they generate a wave of coherence and calm that reaches beyond the individual, influencing the energy in the Field. This energy can impact people and events around them. We have mentioned the power of group heart coherence in Chapter 2. The interconnected energy of people raising their frequencies is hard to describe; you must experience it to believe. I'll admit that I never imagined it could feel so tangible until I immersed myself in a group meditation. The energy is palpable, feels electric, and is not limited to people being physically present in the same space. Remarkably, the effects can be just as strong when participants are in different locations, even on opposite sides of the world.

I've witnessed this firsthand through distant healings where groups focus their energy on others, often with extraordinary results. The feedback from those receiving these healings has been astounding, affirming the reality of these shared energetic experiences. And it's not just anecdotal; numerous studies have explored the measurable effects of group meditations, including reduced crime rates, decreased stress levels and increased feelings of peace and coherence within communities.

Group energy can amplify the sense of connection and deepen the experience. When people come together and tune into the same frequency, they can create a lasting resonance that lingers in the space, elevating its energy long after they've left. So if nobody in your life is interested in meditating with you, perhaps you could join a group – feel it for yourself.

In one well-documented event in 1993, around 4,000 Transcendental Meditation practitioners gathered in Washington, D.C., with a shared intention to reduce crime in the city. During the meditation period, researchers observed a significant drop in violent crime rates; some studies estimate it to be as much as 23%. The findings were surprising, as the decrease occurred despite other factors that typically increase crime in summer.

Another striking example of group meditation was a large-scale meditation event in the early 2000s, where approximately 7,000 participants came together with a shared intention — to increase global peace. Their collective meditation focused on reducing violence and fostering harmony on a worldwide scale. Researchers monitoring the event observed a noticeable decrease in global tensions during this period, suggesting that the power of synchronised intention may extend far beyond the individuals involved.

Studies like these suggest that collective meditation doesn't just benefit the participants; it creates a ripple effect in the Field, influencing others and generating harmony. This phenomenon offers a glimpse of the power that unified thought and intention can have when directed through a shared focus, underscoring the potential of our energy to shape the world around us.

Quiet Fields - The Power of Global Sleep Times

If you are wondering what time you should meditate, any time of the day works; you should do it anytime you can. Many teachers recommend doing so first thing in the morning. The reasoning for morning meditation is that your brain transitions from slower brain wave states, such as delta and theta experienced during sleep, into more active states, like alpha and beta. During this transition, your mind is naturally more receptive and calmer, making it an ideal meditation time. Morning meditations also help set a positive tone for the day ahead.

While there are definite benefits to starting your day with meditation, I've discovered something no one seems to be discussing. This discovery began when I noticed that my deepest meditations consistently happen between coming home from work and heading to Pilates, usually around 3 p.m. Even though these sessions are quick and often rushed, they are always the deepest compared to meditations at other times of the day. At first, I thought this was just my personal experience, but then I started wondering if there could be a more significant reason behind this.

It led me to an insight I haven't heard anyone else explore: the idea that the best time to meditate might not be when your brain waves are in the right state. There might be another factor.

This idea came to me one day when I was listening to a podcast, and they mentioned the concept of meditating when the Field around you is quiet. That's when it hit me. If the Field exists beyond time and space, and the collective energy of the world influences it, then what if the most potent time to meditate isn't just when it's quiet around me—but when it's quiet across the entire world?

This realisation sparked a deep dive into the concept. I wondered if the global collective energy, shaped by the rhythms of waking and sleeping populations, could influence the Field. With the help of AI, we set out to explore this idea. We started by looking at where most of the world's population is located across different time zones and putting it into percentages. Then, we calculated the average times people are asleep in those regions, factoring in cultural differences and typical schedules. From there, we established when 80-85% of the population is in deep sleep. The calculation was **Universal Time (UTC), 4 am to 6 am.**

For me, living in Australia, that UTC converts to between 2 pm and 4 pm AEST. That was the exact time I was having my most profound meditations. This time is when many parts of the world, especially heavily populated regions like Europe and Asia, are asleep or just waking up. I realised I had been tapping into a quieter, less energetically crowded field. So, if you're an Aussie, I encourage you to try meditating between 2 pm and 4 pm AEST. Other regions that could still be awake are the west coast of the U.S., Pacific Islands, Southeast Asia and parts of East Asia.

Changing your meditation time could be a powerful window to tap into the stillness of the Field, so do a time conversion from the UTC mentioned and see if you can experiment with meditating at that time. It could make for a fascinating experience.

I encourage you to experiment with meditation to see what works for you: time, location or different styles. As we leave the quiet of global sleep cycles behind, it's time to dive into the rich tapestry of real-life meditation experiences. Each one is beautifully unique, reminding us there's no 'good' or 'bad' meditation, only your personal journey unfolding perfectly.

Real-Life Stories from Regular Meditators

Now, we reach the part of the book I'm most excited about! Why? It's precisely what I wish I could have read when I first started meditating, and honestly, even now, I'm still fascinated by hearing people's stories. Meditation journeys are deeply personal, yet we rarely get a glimpse into the raw, unfiltered experiences of others.

What follows are six incredible stories from people I know personally, each sharing their unique meditation journey. I've asked them to be unfiltered, with no holding back. These stories are honest, inspiring, and sometimes unexpected. These people come from different backgrounds and are aged between 20 and 60. That is the beauty of meditation: it suits everyone and is free. Most of these people found it difficult to put their experiences into words, so I am very grateful that they all pushed through, and I am sure you will be, too. Get ready to dive into meditation's real, unpolished magic as seen through different people's perspectives and experiences.

MICHELLE W

At the beginning of 2024, my father passed away, leaving me in a deeply low emotional state. I had recently started taking antidepressants when my acupuncturist recommended a book called Letting Go by David R. Hawkins. Reading this book sparked a shift in my perspective, opening my mind to the possibility that there was more to life than the limited thinking and reality I had been experiencing. This marked the beginning of my personal development journey. The following recommendation I received was to try meditation, which led me to explore the teachings of Dr. Joe Dispenza.

Dr Joe teaches that our personality creates our personal reality. Our personality is how we think, act and feel. I knew I needed to change my personality to create a new and better reality. Following Dr Joe's teachings, I started setting the 5 am alarm each morning for meditation. I have tried relaxation meditations on YouTube but have not been able to get into a meditative state like Dr Joe's meditations. I find that an hour of meditation each morning helps my day start on the right note. It allows me to calm my mind and reduce the constant stream of thoughts that used to flood my head. The feeling of inner calm is so lovely that it motivates me to wake up early to meditate each morning. Fast forward to now, it has become an addiction I can't imagine living without. No matter what, I do my meditations.

This practice gives me a sense of calm throughout the day, allowing me to handle situations more effectively. I am more self-aware and able to stay present, rather than being stuck in a constant loop of thoughts like, 'What did I say to that person yesterday?' 'They must think I'm...' or 'What's going to happen when...'. While I still catch myself slipping into these thought patterns, the difference now is that I am aware enough to gently bring myself back and focus on what I'm doing in the moment.

Meditation has had an overall positive impact on my life; I was only on the antidepressants for eight days and have not for one minute considered going back on them. My brain secretes feel-good chemicals now, and I have no doubt this is a response to my daily meditation ritual. I am now so grateful for all the blessings in my life; the cup is half full instead of half empty. When fear and worry creep in (as they often do — I have two teenage daughters and have always been an overprotective mother), or when I wake up in the middle of the night with something on my mind that stirs negative thoughts, I place my hands over my heart and simply feel. This practice brings me fully into the present moment, making it impossible to focus on anything else. My new mantra is: 'The past is the past, and the present is a gift.'

On a more personal note, I was raised Catholic and later developed strong Christian beliefs. For a long time, whenever I encountered anything related to spirituality, energy or meditation, I would immediately shut it down, believing it wasn't aligned with God. Since I started on this journey, I can say that I now feel closer to God than I ever have. I have realised that God is not outside me, looking down and judging everything

I do wrong. This belief held me back for many years. I know now that the Kingdom of God lives within me.

PETER W

I initially decided to start meditating to lower my blood pressure, as I was determined not to rely on medication. I began with short 15-minute meditations on Spotify. Nine months ago, I committed to attending a Dr Joe Dispenza retreat with my wife, which required a lot of preparation through online education. As part of this, I started practising his meditations daily. These meditations were much longer and more immersive than anything I'd done before. These days, I find that I can no longer do short meditations; I need longer ones. Waking up every morning with Michelle and committing to the work has been a transformative journey. In addition to meditating, I began listening to books and podcasts from various teachers, all centred around consciousness. I found myself diving down the rabbit hole of life, becoming resolute in my determination to take control of my own destiny.

To this day, I haven't missed a day of meditation. My main focus has been on awaiting a mystical experience. Only now, as I write this, are things starting to happen in my breathwork. I started to notice some unique things happening with my body. During my breathwork to activate my pineal gland just this week, I began experiencing strange involuntary movements, first on one side, then the other. It felt like my arm was reaching for something on the floor, and my leg was lifting vertically. It's bizarre, but I wasn't scared. Interestingly, as soon as I focus on it, the sensations disappear. I've also heard distant voices during these moments. I can't wait to see what happens next. Beyond the mystical experiences, I've noticed significant changes in my external life. Although I was only focused on the mystical, some surprising changes were starting to happen that I hadn't planned. For instance, I no longer have road rage and things that used to bother me just don't bother me anymore; I just let them go; it's not worth spoiling my peace of mind. This has become my new way of life, and I'm excited about the future and for my manifestations to come to fruition when the time is right.

TOM D

I've been experimenting with different methods, such as Wim Hof breathing, on and off for a few years. I read The Power of Now a few years ago, which gave me my initial eye-opening experiences. Still, meditation didn't fully resonate until about 10 months ago, when I began meditating consistently.

I meditate daily, with sessions ranging from 15 minutes to 1 hour, occasionally extending to 1 hour and 30 minutes when I feel called to dive deeper.

I primarily use Joe Dispenza's guided meditations, which have been transformative in helping me connect with deeper states of consciousness. At times, I also enjoy listening to binaural beats and focusing on my breath, allowing myself to simply be present in the moment.

I would like to describe a profound mystical experience I had. It all started the day before the event; I was in Townsville for work and had free time before my flight back to the Gold Coast. I decided to explore a hill in the middle of Townsville. As I sat there, I focused on connecting mentally with the landscape, contemplating the interconnectedness of the land, the energy of the place and everything around me. This deep connection with nature felt grounding and likely prepared me for the intense experience I would have the next day.

The following day, in staying with the nature connection theme, I began with a morning surf session, followed by a walk through a Japanese-inspired garden. Later, around 3 pm, I had some blue lotus tea, I felt a gentle body high and a deep sense of connection. That evening, I sat by a fire near the water, gazing at the moon and feeling profoundly connected to everything around me. It wasn't until around 11 pm, while watching a movie with friends that I was suddenly overwhelmed by a pulse of energy. Everything blurred, and an uncontrollable grin spread across my face. Moments later, the energy returned, and I knew I needed to meditate. I went to my room, put on a meditation, and was immediately immersed in the experience. Throughout the session, I felt intense energy bursts that lifted my chest. My breathing shifted rhythmically in patterns that felt completely involuntary. My watch recorded my heart rate between 90 and 135 bpm during the session, a dramatic shift from my usual resting heart rate of 45 bpm. At times, the energy felt as though it was moving through me, guiding my body's rhythms. As the meditation deepened, my hands moved involuntarily into mudras (yoga-like hand gestures), and I began speaking in a language I had never heard before. Fully aware of what was happening, I chose not to focus on it, understanding that giving it too much attention could end the experience. I visualised different life scenarios, seeing how each path could lead me to exactly where I wanted to be. These scenarios felt as real as my current material reality. Each time I delved deeply into one, I was 'zoomed' back out to myself. In those moments, I knew that everything I needed was within me. I just needed to connect to my heart. I realised that spending time in nature is vital for me and that this connection is key to unlocking my potential.

The next day, I shared my experience with Kylie, who revealed that many other meditators have reported similar occurrences, including spontaneous movements and speaking unknown languages. She found numerous accounts in a Facebook group of meditators describing the phenomenon. Intrigued, I researched further and discovered 'light language,' a language of higher consciousness. It felt as though I had uncovered something deeply meaningful, something that had been within me all along. It was one of the most profound moments of my life, leaving me with a sense of clarity, love and connection.

Besides the above mystical event, my body often reacts uniquely during meditation. I experience an uncontrollable smile or grin during moments of intense energy. I sometimes feel an upward pull in my chest or find my hands moving involuntarily into mudras. These responses feel like natural expressions of energy moving through me.

I have to say that meditation has profoundly altered my perception of life and my connection to the world around me. My nervous system feels more balanced, and I experience a sense of calm and clarity that stays with me throughout my days. Synchronicities have become an everyday occurrence, happening multiple times daily in ways that seem almost unfathomable. A recent example illustrates this beautifully. While at work, a fly landed on me in my upstairs office, where I'd never seen a fly before. I shooed it away, but 30 seconds later, it landed on me again. This caught my attention, and I decided to let it be. The next day, I listened to a podcast where the host discussed the art of contemplation and shared an example of signs appearing in daily life. His specific example? A fly landing on you, being flicked away, and returning — a reminder from your guides to pause, be present, and reflect. Moments like this have become so frequent that they no longer shock me. Instead, they fill me with gratitude and awe. They're beautiful reminders of the interconnectedness of all things and the incredible potential we tap into when we align with our inner selves and reconnect with the source of all that is.

If I could give tips for those starting in meditation, they would be:

1. Start with a guide: Use guided meditations, like Joe Dispenza's, to help structure your practice.
2. Be open: Trust the process. Every experience, whether subtle or intense, is valuable.

3. Stay consistent: Meditate daily, even for just a few minutes, to build the habit.
4. Embrace nature: Spending time in nature has profoundly enhanced my meditation journey.

My final thoughts on meditation are that it is an invitation to explore your inner world and connect with the deeper aspects of life. Each experience, whether ordinary or extraordinary, offers valuable lessons and insights. Trust yourself, lean into the practice, and know that love and connection are at the core of it all.

ANDREW S

My meditation journey began 30 years ago, during my 20th year on this planet. I had a deep desire to learn the art of meditation, and fate led me to a remarkable woman. She was well-known for helping people navigate health and life challenges with a beautiful spiritual approach to everything she did. I remember her presence vividly, unlike anyone I'd ever encountered. She exuded a calmness and warmth that immediately drew me in. Intrigued, I asked her to teach me how to meditate. In just a few training sessions, she seemed to have an uncanny ability to tune into my preferences, even choosing the perfect meditation music for me, a soundtrack I couldn't get enough of. I used her meditation approach, which was pretty basic, just to focus on the space around me and to visualise my desired life. I started focusing on creating the opportunities and a life that I desired. Little did I know how quickly my desires would manifest in the coming months and years. I have never looked back since meeting that lady so many years ago.

When I started meditating, I worked in hospitality as a waiter, but on weekends, my love was racing my bicycle, and I was pretty good at it, too. Life was pretty simple at 21; I had two goals: one was to race in

Europe, and the other was to change careers. Within months, I achieved outstanding results in my cycling. I received an opportunity to race in Germany, semi-professionally, even though I didn't speak German. Once in Germany, I managed to find myself a part-time job as a bicycle mechanic. I was living my dreams. Coincidence? No.

Fast track a couple of years, and I was living in California; I continued on my spiritual path and couldn't get enough of spiritual books, texts and many teachings. I was guided by my fascination and curiosity, which led to my decision to study acupuncture in Australia the following year after one last season of racing in Germany. I had worked out by now that the more often I meditated, the calmer I felt in my outer world, and the more synchronicities appeared.

I continued the work in my 30s and was still meditating fairly regularly and learning other methodologies like chanting, immersion in joy and love, contemplation, men's retreats, vision quests, sweat lodges and breath techniques. Yep, I was probably considered a bit of a hippy back then because that kind of stuff wasn't very popular.

Skip forward to my forties, and I was starting to really master my skills in concentrating and tuning in to the Field around me. I found this one of my most difficult steps and only really mastered it by this stage in my life (yes, I know, it took a long time). I was now using longer and more disciplined styles of meditation based on techniques and training from many teachers. I started to learn meditation and philosophy with Kadampa Buddhism and then attended regular meditation retreats with the Buddhist monks. The primary methods used were meditating on the breath, mental techniques and mantras.

For the past seven or eight years, I have been studying the work of Dr Joe Dispenza, reading all his books, and attending four of his retreats. His work has taken me to another level. I have had quite a lot of supernatural experiences, and the synchronicities I have experienced are extraordinary.

What I know for sure now is this omnipresent field gives us a feeling that awakens our body's dormant senses and allows us to tune into it. I would describe the feeling of being pulled and drawn in like a magnetic field. I know that everyone has the ability to feel and experience this. You just have to put the work in and commit to regular meditations. It took me many years to get to a state of deep immersion.

These days, I have many wonderful experiences during my meditations, and I can stay in the Field for hours if I choose to. More often than not, I am immersed in a feeling of love, peace and harmony that nourishes me from within. This feeling creates a space for extraordinary, even supernatural, experiences to occur — of which I have had many. In my meditations, I have encountered many beings from other dimensions and often find myself in beautiful and fascinating places. The beings I meet are benevolent and loving; some communicate messages to me, while others just remain present in my Field. I believe they are there to support or observe me on my journey. After meditating for so long, these experiences have become so natural that I rarely feel the need to share them or reflect on them afterwards. Writing this extract has been challenging, as it feels like describing an ingrained part of my life. I suppose it would be like asking someone to articulate the air they breathe, an essential yet often unnoticed act.

Along with creating a calm, nourishing outer world, I also use meditation as a tool to heal the past and overcome obstacles. The main tools I use for this healing work are based on Dr David Hawkins' 'letting go' technique. This technique is designed to move suppressed emotions out of the unconscious mind. What replaces these negative emotions is joy and love that I can feel flowing from my heart. The technique is simple: feel it, stay with it, don't analyse or judge it and just let it be there until it fades away. I did this work for a four-year period in meditations and outside meditations.

Meditation is a beautiful and almost addictive part of my life, and I recommend it to everyone.

DR MARK M

I have been practising meditation and energy work for decades. I meditate daily, sometimes multiple times a day, depending on what's unfolding in my life. My practice blends beautifully — Reiki meditation for energy alignment, Dzogchen for abiding in the natural state of awareness and Vipassana to observe sensations and cultivate mindfulness. Each technique offers unique insights but also weaves into a cohesive whole over time.

I've been practising Reiki for 36 years as a Reiki Master, which has been a profound journey of energy healing and connection. Alongside that, I've been a Dzogchen practitioner for 33 years, delving deeply into the non-dual nature of the mind. My Vipassana and Insight Meditation practice spans 35 years, bringing clarity, mindfulness and insight into my daily life.

In regards to the mystical, meditation has revealed moments of profound stillness and unity — where the boundaries of self and other dissolve entirely. There have been times when colours, light and energy flows became almost tangible, a visceral reminder of the interconnected nature of everything. And then, there are simpler moments: an overwhelming sense of love or deep, abiding peace.

In regards to how my body reacts in meditation, sometimes it is completely still in perfect alignment with the energy flowing through. Other times, there are twitches or spontaneous movements as energy blocks release. Reiki, especially, can cause subtle vibrations or warmth as healing takes place.

Meditation has completely transformed my life. My health feels more resilient, and my nervous system is far more regulated, even in challenging situations. Synchronicities are frequent — meeting the right people, receiving answers when needed or life unfolding in surprisingly harmonious ways. I often feel guided by something larger than myself.

My tips for beginner meditators would be to start small and be gentle with yourself. A few minutes a day can make a big difference. Consistency is more important than perfection. Experiment with techniques until you find one that feels natural. And trust the process — even when it feels challenging, you're growing in ways you might not immediately see.

My final thought is to not be afraid but to embrace the 'weird' or mystical aspects of meditation. It's a deeply personal journey, and everyone's path will be different. Honour your unique experiences, and remember, the most profound growth often happens in the quiet, everyday moments of practice.

JAYE M

I have been meditating on and off since I was 21 years old. However, I stepped it up a notch and started taking it seriously when I was introduced to Dr Joe Dispenza's work. Like many, through his teachings, I was able to expand the time and depth of my meditations, and it opened my mind. Now, I meditate daily for about 15-30 minutes and try to complete longer ones as much as I can. The long meditations are where the magic happens, moving into a deep meditative state where the nagging conscious mind is put aside, and I am relieved from constant thought.

Meditation, for me, has brought a new perspective on what it is to feel, not with the traditional five senses but from within. I can tap into this feeling that is usually drowned out by the external, ever-stimulating world. Before meditation, I never realised how much of the day I was switched on, tuned into every bell and ping from the external environment in a hypnotic, reactive manner — often subconsciously searching for gratifications. Meditation has allowed me to experience internal gratification, and I feel far richer and more fulfilled than I do in the external environment.

In many meditations, even after only practising for less than a year, I am now able to elicit an incredible feeling of bliss and ecstasy throughout my whole body and being. This feeling is a product of reconnecting with Source, the omnipresent energetic lifeforce from which all living things emanate. This life force is something that we lose connection with through our conditioned, stressful lifestyles.

The power of meditation as a vehicle for manifesting abundance through connecting to Source has been indisputable for me, even in my first year alone. As soon as I learned the ropes of quieting my mind and creating feelings of gratitude and love during meditation, one of the first things I began to do was to manifest finding the love of my life.

In Dr. Joe's work, he teaches you to create a specific intention for what you want to manifest and, during meditation, to move into a state of gratitude as if you already have that thing. With plans to move to Amsterdam the following year, my intention was to meet a Dutch girl in Amsterdam who would be the love of my life. After meditating on this for a couple of months, I had a very strange experience. One night, after a deep meditation where I specifically focused on feeling all the emotions of what it would be like to meet her, fall in love, and live in that future state of gratitude, I fell asleep still thinking about her and how amazing life would be. The following day, while working, I checked my phone and saw a message from a friend who lived interstate and had been travelling around Europe. He wrote: 'Dude, do yourself a favour and check your Instagram.'

On Instagram, I found a message from a beautiful girl I had recently seen on a dating app. I'd followed her but hadn't taken any action. Typical. My friend had met this girl during a night out, and my name came up in their conversation when she noticed we had mutual followers. In his message, he added: 'I might have set you up on a little date when she gets back. Bonus: she's Dutch.' That day, she and I began messaging back and forth, and with each exchange, it became increasingly clear how well we got along. At the end of our conversation, in a message, she mentioned she had just landed at her destination. Can you guess where? ... Amsterdam. It wasn't until several synchronicities unfolded in the following days — too many to include in such a short segment —and the awe and disbelief I felt that everything finally clicked for me.

Starting meditations, particularly lengthy ones, when you are just starting out can be difficult at first. I've had many people that I've introduced meditation to tell me that they can't do it because their brain moves too fast. This is exactly why you should persevere. But it doesn't have to be hard. Starting with and being consistent with 15-20 minute daily meditations with a guided program such as Dr Joe's will help you slow your mind easier and easier, sooner than you think. Just commit to 4 weeks of daily practice, and I promise that you will notice the difference. There is no more rewarding feeling than connecting back with Source and your higher self. Take the leap; you have everything to gain.

As you can see from each story, meditation is unique to every individual. The Field offers precisely what each person needs in the moment, tailoring the experience to their journey. What's truly remarkable is that these people are just like you and me, living their lives, facing their challenges, and tapping into something profound. Through meditation, they've discovered their unique superpowers. Whether clarity, healing, manifesting dreams, or simply finding peace in the chaos, these stories show what's possible when we connect with the Field. The potential isn't reserved for a chosen few; it's available to all of us. If they can do it, so can you. I've watched so many people change their lives through meditation, and I think it should be a non-negotiable thing, like brushing your teeth. We will step out of our inner world for the next chapter and consider our bodies.

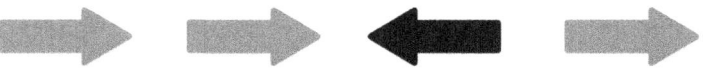

CHAPTER 10

BIOHACKS FOR THE BODY

A fancy term for little changes you can make to take care of your body like it deserves.

There's a ton of information about biohacking, but it's a topic that must be addressed. Why? Because you can't work on your spiritual and emotional self while you're sitting on your butt, eating packaged chemical-laden food, inhaling toxins, skipping sleep, bathing in EMF and slathering yourself and your home with more toxins. Let's be honest; your body deserves better than that!

Writing this chapter was a challenge because, with my background in healthcare and passion for herbal medicine, there was so much I wanted to include. I had to leave many ideas on the editing floor and remind myself to keep things simple. Having experience in both conventional and natural medicine, I can't help but feel that our approach to healthcare is often backwards. The focus should be on prevention and addressing root causes rather than waiting for symptoms to appear and masking them with 'band-aid' treatments. Don't get me wrong, conventional medicine is incredible for acute care and emergencies. However, when it comes to chronic issues and mental illnesses, it's clear that something isn't working because it's getting worse rather than better. The solution lies in empowering individuals to take control of their bodies inside and out.

I am passionate about using herbs and natural remedies to nourish my body — taking them as needed or when intuition calls. What I love about herbs is their innate synergy with the body. Using the whole plant enables them to work across multiple systems, supporting holistic well-being. The world of herbs is so vast that it could easily fill an entire book. If you want to learn about this topic, there are some people I can recommend: Barbara O'Neil, David Avocado Wolfe, Zach Bush M.D, Mason Hutchinson and Thomas Easley, to name a few.

Why look after your body? Some argue, 'If I'm an eternal being, I might as well live however I want.' WRONG. Your body, whether you think of it as your vessel, meat suit, or fancy biological spaceship, needs to be treated with respect. You also want to have the best quality of life possible. It's the foundation of everything you're trying to accomplish in *Opposite World*. If you want to thrive, not just survive, giving your body the cleanest and healthiest environment is non-negotiable. What is the point of doing all the hard work on your emotional body if you don't look after the physical body?

But don't worry, I won't tell you to throw out everything in your pantry or move to a mountaintop. Let's keep it simple: I'm all about moderation and doing the best you can most of the time.

I'll share some easy, practical biohacks that you can add to your life to make a big difference. Everyone's body is unique, so this isn't medical advice; it is simple, easy, and free lifestyle changes. Throughout this book, we have already mentioned some, like being in nature and meditating. All the suggestions in this chapter are just what I do regularly, and I'm sure you'll find a few that resonate with you and easily fit into your life.

Simple 'Free' Daily Biohacks

GROUNDING

Grounding, also called earthing, is basically just putting your bare feet or body on the Earth. No, this is not a woo-woo, hippy myth that gives excuses for not wearing shoes. I admit that I used to think this, too. I know now that it's scientifically proven to benefit us. Why? The Earth's negatively charged electrons balance the electrical charge in your body. As we are energetic beings, some environments can create an excess of positive charges, which lead to imbalances in our bodies and the earth can remedy this.

Benefits: Grounding helps reduce inflammation, improve sleep, and regulate biological rhythms, all of which are essential for good health.

Grounding is essential to maintaining balance and well-being when engaging in energy work, such as deep meditation and breathwork. While these practices can elevate your energy and expand your awareness, staying connected to your body and the earth's stabilising energy is equally important. Grounding helps anchor you in the present moment, preventing feelings of disorientation or imbalance that can sometimes arise with intense spiritual practices. Think of it as creating a strong foundation, allowing you to explore higher realms while staying rooted and supported in your physical self.

There is plenty of information, books and studies on grounding. At a minimum, try to put your feet on the earth for a period of time every day.

SUNGAZING AND THE SUN

I discovered sungazing three years ago, and now I notice when I haven't done it for a few days. What is it? Isn't looking at the sun harmful? Yes and no. If you look at the sun within an hour of sunrise and sunset, it's good for you; outside that small window, it's not so good.

When the sun is low on the horizon, the light is softer, less intense and rich in specific wavelengths that enrich the body and mind. The harmful UV and blue light are filtered out at these times so you won't damage your eyes. Within sunrise and sunset, the light is rich in infrared wavelengths. Infrared, as many know, will penetrate the skin and eyes, which promotes cellular repair and energy production. There are many benefits to sungazing, like your emotions; it is excellent for your mood, as the light can boost your serotonin levels. It is also great for regulating your circadian rhythm, as exposure to this light tells your body when sleep and awake times are. At sunset, sungazing will help produce melatonin for sleep; at sunrise, it will help produce cortisol for energy.

Sungazing is also good for the eyes. In Greek mythology, the sun holds significant symbolism. There is a story about sungazing restoring Queen Merope's eyesight after her father blinded her. It is pretty interesting if you go down a rabbit hole on eyesight and sungazing. For instance, in 1920, William Horatio Bates, an ophthalmologist, published a book based on his findings called *The Perfect Sight Without Glasses*. He rebelled against wearing spectacles, and it seems he was considered controversial for this. His book lays out various techniques; one was sungazing for your eyesight. Not long after his book was published, Bates went missing for years and was eventually found by his wife but had no memory of his past — a mystery that remains unexplained. I'll leave that one for you to ponder. I wish I had sun gazed from a young age; perhaps I wouldn't need reading glasses today.

In the early 1900s, sunglasses were introduced to the masses, and Hollywood stars turned them into essential fashion items for everyone, encouraging the fear of light. But where is science today, more than 100 years later? We still wear glasses and contact lenses, and sunglasses are still a fashion statement. The advice not to stare at the sun with the naked eye still stands strong. I still get surprised when I mention sungazing and people say, 'Oh no, you can't look at the sun'. While mostly true, it's never taught about specific times of the day when it is safe and beneficial. Ironically, some eye conditions are treated with therapies that activate near-infrared light (Albini & Riva, 2020).

Sungazing can take a while to get used to. Start by looking at the sun for a few seconds and gradually increase your gaze to a minute. Experienced sungazers can do it for up to 15 minutes, but you need to build up to that over a long period of time.

It's fun; give it a go. I especially love doing it in public because the looks you get from people are priceless. I also use it as a travel hack when going to different time zones; it helps with jet lag by allowing your body to adjust its circadian rhythm.

Another powerful way to align with natural light cycles is to limit blue light exposure after sunset. While sungazing taps into the benefits of natural sunlight during the day, reducing artificial blue light at night helps support your circadian rhythm and promotes restorative sleep. Simple, cost-free actions like dimming lights or avoiding screens in the evening can make a noticeable difference. Although options like blue light-blocking glasses and specialised light bulbs are available, they involve additional costs, and our focus here is on free biohacks.

Don't you always feel so much better when the sun is shining? That's because the sun does so much more than brighten the day; it brightens you, too. While on the subject of the sun, sungazing isn't its only health benefit. Most people know the sun's role in producing vitamin D, but there's more to its magic. When sunlight reaches your eyes, it stimulates the pineal gland to produce serotonin, the 'feel-good' hormone that boosts your mood during the day. Later, this serotonin transforms into melatonin at night, helping you sleep. Outdoor sunlight amplifies these effects, making it far more potent than indoor light. The pineal gland, often known to be mystical for its role in meditation and higher states of consciousness, has so much untapped potential. But let's save that for the next book or retreat.

To wrap up this conversation about the sun, it's worth noting that recommendations for sun exposure vary widely. The challenge lies in balancing the need for protection from the sun's harsher rays with the undeniable health benefits of sunlight. As with most things in life, the middle ground seems like the wisest choice: protect yourself during the peak, harsh sunlight hours (avoiding chemical-laden sunscreens that can do more harm than good) and soak up the sun's magical, less harmful rays during shorter periods of the day. The key is mindful moderation.

My Biohacking Rituals

I chose grounding and sungazing as the main topics to explore and would love to discuss more. Instead, I will list what I do regularly, and you can choose what suits you best. We all have different bodies, so don't take this as medical advice.

- Herbs — I cycle of and on many, find what's right for you
- Eliminate toxin exposure in my food, skincare, haircare and household products. Tip: use the Yuka app (it will change the way you look at everything)
- Intermittent and extended water fasting
- Exercise daily
- Declutter your space
- Clean, chemical-free water — Our whole-house water is filtered. Depending on where you live, check what is in your tap water. I also add lemon, bicarbonate soda, electrolytes, or occasionally apple cider vinegar to my morning water.
- Cold exposure — activates that brown fat
- Infrared sauna
- Red light therapy
- Weekly detoxing (I change this around often, but examples include taking heavy metal removal herbs, charcoal and a bath with magnesium, bi-carb, pine needle and bentonite clay)
- Parasite cleansing
- Mitigate EMF (don't sleep near your phone or put it on flight mode)
- Nasal breathing

- Holistic oral care — oil pulling (I use coconut oil)
- Manage gut health
- Drink fluids away from food
- Sleep 8 hours per night
- Acupuncture
- Meditate everyday
- MCT Oil in my coffee each morning
- Everything in moderation

We have listed many options here, so choose three and commit to them. Try to do some of these while you do any of your current habits so that it doesn't feel like an effort. Perhaps you already go for nature or beach walks some days. You could combine this walk with watching the sunrise and taking off your shoes.

Your soul chose this body to have your human experience, so look after it.

If you need to be held accountable, write down three biohacks that resonate with you. I will commit to using these three biohacks daily, starting today.

1. _____
2. _____
3. _____

Once your new habits become so second nature that skipping them feels as strange as leaving the house without pants, it's time to add a few more. And don't stress if life happens and you miss a day or a week. If you turn it into a chore, you'll likely abandon ship faster than a bad diet. Aim for the 80/20 rule: 80% of the time, nourish and nurture your body, and the other 20%, give yourself a break. Have that pizza, skip that workout, or sleep in — you're human, not a robot. I've had my fair share of undisciplined moments, but I remind myself that my overall effort counts. And guilt? We are not doing guilt; we've learnt that low-frequency emotions can make us sick.

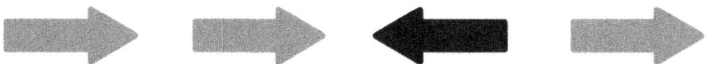

CHAPTER 11

REALIGNING RELATIONSHIPS AS YOU TRANSFORM

Yes, growth can be a bit awkward sometimes.

Embracing Change While Others Stay the Same

As you grow and evolve in different areas of life, you may encounter people in your world who remain the same, and the contrast can feel challenging. Such differences can make your transition to the external world seem isolating or unsettling. Many people go through this, yet it's a topic that often goes unspoken. Please feel reassured that you're not alone on this journey. I get it and hope to offer some helpful advice.

I have been using the term *Opposite World* for years. It was almost my coping mechanism to understand why I often take a different mindset than most people. It was my way of adding humour when feeling like the minority. We frequently hear about incredible stories of transformation, healing and manifestation during an awakening or transformation, but we rarely hear about the other side of it. People can feel isolated and feel like they are living in a completely different world. Well, they are living in *Opposite World*. Many describe it as feeling as if you used to live in a bubble and are suddenly aware of things they had overlooked before. At first, this new awareness can feel so unfamiliar that some wish they could return to the comfortable oblivion of unawareness. However, over time, they adapt, settle into their new reality, and learn to appreciate their transformation deeply. It's much like introducing a fish to a new tank; at first, it needs time to adjust, floating in its plastic bag, but eventually, it embraces its new expansive world.

As you grow and are on the path to awakening, you start feeling more amazing and whole, and naturally, you will want everyone around you to feel the same joy and transformation. Honestly, the reality is that many people resist change; it is hard for them to see outside their programming. You may even find that your growth may provoke discomfort in others as it triggers something deep inside them that they are not ready to face and may never be. As you grow and shine your light brighter, you will also have to develop a thick skin because you will be going against the norm, or I call it going against 'normie world'. Your growth may lead to some awkwardness or criticism. In *Opposite World*, we experience this often but brush it off and don't take it personally. We know we are doing the best we can for ourselves. When you are judged or ridiculed by others, remember to stay anchored and true to yourself, don't doubt yourself, and keep shining your light because otherwise, it will lower your frequencies. The unfortunate truth is that some people may like you better when you are weaker because it makes them feel better. At the end of the day, everyone has their perspective that they believe to be true, which must be respected.

You don't need to explain or justify yourself to people about your transformations, and you don't need to argue your points or prove that you are right and they are wrong. Keep in mind that arguing is just a battle of egos wanting to be correct.

I have some advice: this took me quite some time to learn. The most important thing you need to know is that you can never change or fix someone. People can only fix themselves and possibly don't want to or are not ready to. Know that everyone is exactly where they are supposed to be. Don't judge anyone; know that we are all at different levels of consciousness. Instead of preaching to people, live the best way you can and hope they can sense your radiance. As you transform and raise your frequency levels, people around you may also; it's a natural, energetic transition. You may find certain people are drawn to you and want to ask questions; of course, these people are the ones you are supposed to help, but you can only offer advice to the people who ask for it. As Michael Jackson says in Man in the Mirror, *if you want to make the world a better place, take a look at yourself and make a change.* Think of it this way: your love can be the bridge that helps others connect to the Field — whether energetically or simply by embodying your highest self. The more deeply you know yourself, the more you naturally inspire transformation in those around you.

I want you to remember this. People can only hear information that matches their frequency. I'll say that again because it is important: '**People can only hear information that matches their frequency**'. You'll be banging your head against the wall trying to share your truths with those still stuck in low emotions—fear, unworthiness, and a victim mentality. Programming runs deep, and until a person is prepared to look inside, they cannot see outside their perspective. They feel more comfortable following societal norms. I understand it is hard, but instead of feeling sad or annoyed at them, know that this is where they choose to be for whatever reason; this is where they are supposed to be. If they are people you love, don't judge; love them for who they are. Everything is perfect.

A statement I love from the *Kybalion* is, '**The lips of wisdom are closed, except to the ears of understanding.**' Buddha's teachings also emphasise discernment when sharing spiritual insights, particularly with those who may not be ready to understand or accept them. Both teachings emphasise that you should not push your newfound learnings on people who don't want to or are not ready to hear them. They also reinforce the abovementioned, saying people can only take in information that matches their frequency.

It is not just when you embark on self-transformation that you notice your outer world change. Think of a time when you had a significant life change, such as travelling extensively, moving away from your hometown, or having children. There will always be people in your life that you don't relate to anymore, but you can still love them.

Protect Your Energy

As you begin to raise your frequencies, you will be more sensitive to lower frequencies. Well, at least, that is what I have experienced. You may find people in your life who are energy drainers, and when you are with them, you feel awful. If they are people that you know don't have your best interests at heart, let them go; they cannot stay in your space. **As you grow, there will always be people in your rearview mirror.** If they are not someone you can remove from your life, you can learn to put energy protectors around you. Take a breath and stay in your heart; their energy will not be able to come near or affect you. Higher frequencies will always dominate the lower frequencies. You will naturally find a way to protect your energies because you don't want to return to living out of those lower emotions. You want to live out of your heart. If I encounter people with lower frequencies and cannot physically remove myself from their presence, I visualise a white shield surrounding my body — a field of love. I breathe deeply in and out of my heart; it makes a difference. On the positive side, this practice might even help raise their frequency. They may find themselves feeling lighter or less anxious without knowing why.

Stay on Your Bridge

Stay focused on your dreams; you have worked too hard to drop the ball now. Continue being your own alchemist and spiritual Jedi. If you fall off the bridge for a while, get back on and don't let anything or anyone block your path. Sometimes you feel like you are living on another planet to most people around you. You are starting to be the person you are supposed to be. Don't let that go; stay on your soul's path. Know that your work is changing your timelines and the energy in the Field as a collective. You are helping humanity by giving more love to the Field.

Picture life like this: most of humanity is part of a sweeping wave; they all think the same and do things the same based on societal programming and don't dare to get off the wave. There is immense pressure to conform to popular opinions, trends, and group dynamics. You probably used to be on that wave, but now you feel like you are swimming against it. The general energy of the wave doesn't align with your new values or personal growth. This wave is mighty, and gains strength the more you engage with it. I'll tell you a secret: going in a different direction from this wave is OK. Think of the ocean; what do lifeguards say if you are in a rip? They say, don't fight it; swim parallel to the shore, calm down, and save energy. You can do this in your life: stay grounded and authentic to yourself and refuse to be carried away; this will help you keep your energy and focus intact.

It's okay to ride your unique wave in life; growth often means paddling in the opposite direction to others — stay in your flow. When you resist the pull of the wave, you gain the freedom to chart your unique course, even if it sometimes feels uncertain. The more you practice stepping out of these currents, the more empowered and confident you'll feel in staying true to yourself. Seeing people grounded in who they are is so refreshing, and a bonus is that it's healthy for your body.

A book called *Reality Transurfing* by Vadim Zeland explores this concept well. The book describes the collective as the pendulum. The pendulum is a powerful metaphor for external forces that feed on collective energy, thriving on conflict, drama and attention. Pendulums can represent anything from societal expectations to workplace politics or negative group dynamics. They grow stronger as you engage with them, pulling you into their rhythm and away from your personal growth. The beauty of this concept is its simplicity; ignoring the pendulum robs it of power. You maintain your energy and alignment by consciously choosing not to react or get entangled. This act of detachment allows you to stay true to your path, even when those around you are trapped in their loops of negativity or stagnation.

Think of the pendulum as a force that pulls people into its rhythm. This force thrives on attention and reaction, but here's the empowering part: you don't have to play along. By stepping back and choosing not to engage, you take back control of your energy and focus.

The Power of Saying No

Boundaries are so important, especially when you are working on transformation. You are better off having a much smaller number of people in your life with matching frequencies than many friends who drain you. In *Opposite World*, we don't conform just to fit; we don't care whether people like us or not. There is such power in that feeling; as long as we know we come from love, that is all that matters. What people think about you is not your business, and honestly, most of the time, if you come from love and they judge you, they are really judging themselves. Time is precious. Say no to things you don't want to do, and never fall prey to FOMO (fear of missing out). Please don't rely on validation from anyone; you don't need it; you are running your show. Sit in your silent power. Once you have cleared all your lower emotions, you won't need validation to feel whole. Let's look at this from a spiritual perspective. Your higher self doesn't have to prove itself to anyone and is focused on serving a higher cause for itself and humanity.

In *Opposite World,* we love saying no to things that don't serve us and feel no guilt for doing so. So, find your people, your like-minded tribe that nourishes you, and stick with them. Cherish your alone time because that is when real change happens.

Moving Beyond Generational Limits

I guess there is more to this conversation, and that is our family in this life. For whatever reason, our souls were drawn to the bodies we are in. Some of the blocked emotions or beliefs discussed in this book may stem from generational programming, and who knows how long they date back. It's our karma for this life. You may come from a line of people stuck in survival mode or with a victim mentality, a scarcity mindset (we discussed this in money mindset); they may harbour emotion suppression or conflict avoidance, resulting in passive communication, and so on. These programs are all outdated, and guess what? You may just be the one chosen to clear them. You have the message by now to always be curious and open and not live a life trapped behind limiting beliefs. You'll never grow if you keep hiding behind these beliefs. Most people would continue to live the same way because the programming is so deep; honestly, they don't even realise it's programming. Or if they do, they don't think it can be changed; they believe this is how it is. You may start to think, what happens if I am no longer loyal to this way of thinking? Will I be ostracised? You may be the first person in your family to start doing this work, and feelings of betrayal may come up either from you or your family. Most people who think outside the programming do feel like outcasts, like the black sheep of the family. Some of you may always have been a non-conformist with your feet heading towards *Opposite World*, and you come across as a rebel. This rebellion has always felt natural; you've tried to conform, but it doesn't feel right.

Know that you are not an outcast but a unicorn in your lineage. It is a gift to think outside the box. By doing this work on yourself, you are cleaning your lineage. You are breaking these negative emotions and thoughts on yourself and future generations. Remember that there is no time and space in the Field. You are clearing emotions from both your historical and future generations. So, if you feel ostracised or get a bit of criticism, silently think to yourself, 'You're welcome'. Lean into your heart and know that most people only dictate what they believe to be true (programming).

I often hear people blame their upbringing for all their issues. Don't blame anyone for your shadows; you'll never know how far back they go. Just get on with healing yourself. Your future generations are rooting for you; they would rather have a clean slate to be born into.

Family bonds can be powerful but aren't always meant to last a lifetime. Sometimes, the people we share blood with are part of our journey for a reason, but not forever. If someone in your family has caused significant pain and continues to do so, it may be that their role in your life was to teach you lessons about resilience, boundaries, or self-love. Perhaps your role in their life was to offer them the same opportunity for growth. Letting go doesn't mean you stop caring or wishing them well. It means you have prioritised your peace and healing. You may find yourself on a different frequency that doesn't match theirs. They would find it uncomfortable to be around you with this mismatched energy. If your relationship with your family is toxic or even unsafe, you can send them love from a distance that says, 'I honour the lessons we've shared, but I choose to move forward in a way that supports my well-being.' Doing so gives you and them the space to grow as it's meant to be.

It's okay to go against the grain in life. Growth often means stepping out of the crowd and standing firm in what feels right. When you resist the pull of the wave or pendulum, you become free to follow your unique path, even if it sometimes feels lonely. True empowerment comes from realising that your energy is yours to direct, not something to be drained by trends, collective chaos, or generational trauma. Be the master of your life, and be proud of it.

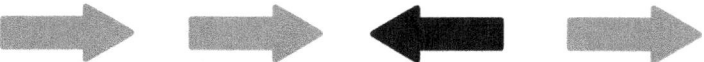

CHAPTER 12

YOUR ACTION BLUEPRINT

Let's integrate all these elements into a cohesive plan and discuss your purpose.

Well done on making it this far in the book. You might find it beneficial to revisit chapters that didn't seem relevant before or even to recap.

Before implementing a tangible plan, I wanted to discuss your purpose. Are you unsure of your purpose or what you really want in life? Do you feel you are supposed to find some magical purpose that was set for you at birth? Don't worry — everything will flow once all the ducks are in a row, and you are comfortable with your current situation. The word 'purpose' gets thrown around often, but what does it mean?

Many feel obligated to discover their single purpose, disheartened by others' apparent fulfilment. For instance, the lady down the road who quit her high corporate job after discovering her highest value (creativity) is now a famous artist. It's not like that for everyone. Finding one's true calling may require time. Rather than searching for your purpose, I believe living a purposeful life is the key. What does that mean? You will live a purposeful and happy life once you align with your values in all areas. Living this way could be the path to finding your 'one purpose' or not; either way, you are happy. The *Course in Miracles* teaches that true happiness comes from embracing your divine nature and releasing illusions. Your divine nature is the most authentic version of you that is living within your values. Return to Chapter 3 to determine your highest value if you haven't already done so. Take a step back, give yourself time, and decide what it is.

Let's see an example of how you can live your life with purpose rather than searching for purpose. Mark's highest value is 'service to others'. Here is a typical day for him. He starts his day by volunteering at a soup kitchen. At work, he spends his afternoon mentoring a colleague. He ends his evening calling a friend who's been going through a tough time. Every action, big or small, reflects his commitment to helping, leaving him feeling deeply fulfilled and purposeful. Although he doesn't say he has found his purpose in the grand scheme of life, he can say he lives a purposeful life and is happy and fulfilled.

Our purpose may not be a treasure to be unearthed but a fluid journey offering different facets of fulfilment. You won't find your purpose until you know who you are — the real you, not the fake persona the world sees. Create distance from your busy life and mind to clear your body of unwanted energetic obstacles and continue to choose love. Your body will then become a transmitter to your higher self. The cleared space will allow light to come in; watch what will begin to emerge. What do I mean by that? You may get messages in your meditation or dreams as words or visions. Synchronicities may appear in your life that you can't ignore. You may develop new talents or old ones you forgot you had. Random opportunities that you least expect may appear. Observe all that seems like random happenings around you. You could miss all these gifts if you don't step back and observe.

While on this ride, find your inner child; what did you love doing when you were young? This may lead you to your purpose; you were much more open back then, closer to your higher self. Meanwhile, appreciate the present, live in the now, and look forward to the future, but don't obsess over finding your purpose. Stay on the bridge and keep clearing the way, even if there's still a little traffic. You don't need to see the end yet — it's on its way. Like driving at night, focus your light on the road ahead. You don't need to see the destination five kilometres away; you know it's there. Keep moving forward, one step (or kilometre) at a time. If you continue to do this work and live in alignment, things will appear when you least expect it. One day, you will say, 'Oh, there it is, that's my purpose!'.

> *The meaning of life is to find your gift, and the purpose of life is to give it away.*
> —Pablo Picasso

~

Your Tangible Plan

Let us recap the book and make some tangible plans. Here is the order of your main focus moving forward.

EVERYTHING COMES FROM THE HEART

I have made this the first point, but it's not a step; it's a new way of living. Everything you do and everything you say comes from the heart. In any situation, ask yourself, 'What would love do?' If you feel annoyed or stressed, stop, close your eyes, breathe, and feel your heart centre.

WHO AM I?

You should have come up with your highest value or values. Write it on a Post-it note, make it your phone's screensaver, or put it somewhere to remind yourself that everything you do must align with this.

RELEASE EMOTIONS

In your day-to-day life, pay close attention to your emotions. Pay attention to what is triggering you. Pay attention to that background feeling in your quiet moments — transmute low-frequency emotions to love. Reread Chapter 4, Unmasking Your Hidden Shadows Within, if necessary.

Continue to release any hidden emotions with the R.E.L.E.A.S.E. tool; use this tool often, every day, or more than that.

THOUGHT SCULPTING

As well as your emotions, pay attention to your thoughts. Those pesky little negative thoughts that think they can rule you — they can't. Practice the tools in the book. It may take a while, but chip away at it, and eventually, the positive way of thinking will become natural.

MEDITATION AND MANIFESTATION

If you want to change your life, learn how to meditate. You can manifest while meditating, but don't make that your only goal; meditation has many other benefits. Once you nail all these steps, what you want will come easily. Start with just five minutes a day and build on that.

BIOHACKS

Don't forget that you need to look after your body. I'm sure you have heard the saying that your body is your temple. Well, it's true.

Claim Your Keys to Unlock a New Life in *Opposite World*

You were offered keys throughout the book; these are listed below. Have you written next to any of them yet? Which ones resonate with you, and which ones would you like to take into your life to live by? All of them are profound if you sit with them. I think of many of them as I go about my days.

Your Life Keys

CHAPTER	🗝	NOTES
The Field	You are always connected—trust and tune in.	
Heart Resilience	Live through the heart.	
Who am I	I see myself in the reflections of others. To change your world, know yourself.	
Life Alignment Tracker	Wholeness starts within – love yourself first, and the rest will fall into place.	
Unmasking the Silent Shadows Within	When I release my shadows, I bring light in.	
Thought Sculpting	The thoughts I choose to focus on shape the life I create.	
Principle of Polarity	Suffering fades when I recognise the polarity within it.	
Be Your Own Alchemist	Miracles only happen when you choose love over fear. Surrender to allow flow.	
Layers of You	We are the universe observing itself through our eyes. We are infinite consciousness having a human experience.	

This book is designed to examine all areas of your life holistically, which means it contains a wealth of information. For that reason, I have devised a way for you to track your progress and hold yourself accountable. Suppose you have your own way of monitoring yourself; great. If you would like an idea, read on.

You could use a simple daily scoring system to measure and reflect on your journey. I call it resilience insurance.

Resilience Insurance

Think of the energy you feed your body and mind daily as stepping stones toward your higher self. Just as food nourishes your body, the energy you nurture within fuels your life force. How you manage and direct this life force determines how you can begin to align with your purpose and measure your personal growth. This is the essence of what I call 'resistance insurance'. It's a strategy to ensure you consistently invest in the energy that moves you closer to your highest potential. It's like keeping track of your meals when you're on a health kick, but this is monitoring how you nourish your thoughts in your internal world.

To give you an idea, imagine that after reading this book, you have promised yourself to work on these. Your goals may be different. This is just an example:

1. Turn your negative thoughts into positive ones.
2. Practice grounding daily.
3. Meditate daily.
4. Challenge your limiting beliefs.

To measure your progress, you can award yourself points at the end of each day. You can also deduct points when your actions or thoughts lower your energy frequency.

Here's how it works:
- **Set a goal:** For example, aim for 20 points by bedtime.
- **Award points for high-frequency actions:** Give yourself two points for every uplifting action or thought.
- **Deduct points for low-frequency actions:** Subtract two points for actions or thoughts that drain your energy.

Example Day
- You wake up after eight hours of restorative sleep, walk barefoot, watch the sunrise, and meditate. Boom! That's 10 points right there.
- You curse someone in traffic and think about how much you dislike your job. Oops! Minus four points.
- Negative thoughts creep in about your health or what others think of you, but you consciously turn them into positive affirmations. Great job! Add two points.
- You choose a chemical-free lunch. Nice choice! Add two more points.
- You genuinely feel happy for a friend's success instead of your usual jealousy. Wonderful! Another two points.

By the time you get home, you've tallied up 12 points and are motivated to get to your 20 points, so you'll probably focus on the last eight points.

Over time, you'll aim to build a 'savings account' of resilience, or resilience insurance. With this bank of high-frequency energy, your body and mind will vibrate so optimally that you'll handle unexpected challenges gracefully and with strength. You may even find after a period that you earn 50 points without even trying because it has become natural. If that is the case, add some more promises to yourself.

Keep a daily record of your points. Over time, this simple system will clearly show where you're thriving and where you could improve. Celebrate your wins and use the insights to focus on areas that need attention. The goal isn't perfection but progress, a steady climb toward a higher vibration and a more resilient you.

FINAL WORDS

Remember the person we talked about at the very start of Chapter 1? That mysterious, powerful person whom you feel drawn to? Guess what? It's you; it's a mirror of who you truly are. The search is over; it was you all along.

My hope for you is that you feel empowered to create your dream life — your little heaven on Earth. Remember to live every day in this new state of love. Apply your new skills daily to overcome life's obstacles. Find joy in everyday moments and get in nature as much as possible. Keep finding the humour in life as you take this journey. Keeping it light will help you stay grounded and resilient, no matter what challenges come your way. Always work on coherence in your heart, mind, and spirit. Remember that anything that takes you away from that will take you away from your higher self.

Live through your heart, learn the opposites of life, love everything, love the bad, the trauma, the darkness, your quirks — love it all. It's a difficult concept to grasp, but as mentioned, suffering only exists when you can't see its polarity. Every night, reflect on how much of your day you lived from your heart. If you closed it, that's ok; just be aware. Any challenges you experience along the way will be worth it.

Spend as many quiet moments in your day as possible to tap into your intuition and always be true to yourself. Your authenticity will grow stronger each day. Follow your truth! Think of truth as a tuning fork to guide you; you don't hear it — you feel it. It's like when you get tingly and goosebumpy when someone speaks because it's the truth. Feel the energy of the truth. Keep finding your truth and be proud of it.

Remember that we are all intuitive mystics. Some of us just have to quiet the noise to tap in. I truly hope you enjoyed the ride. I encourage you to re-read chapters as you evolve and keep this book as your guide to your heart.

It's not goodbye; it's see you soon and see you in the Field.

Jump on our website for free worksheets that align with the book. **www.oppositeworld.org**

This book is just the beginning. My vision extends beyond these pages — learning continues once we step into *Opposite World*. I'd love to hear from you! Let me know which topics resonate most or what you'd like to explore further. Your feedback will help shape what comes next.

If this book sparked new insights, I'd love for you to leave a review. Even a few words would mean the world.

I know you will love your new life in *Opposite World*. Welcome home!

I am so grateful to you all!

Kylie x

ABOUT THE AUTHOR

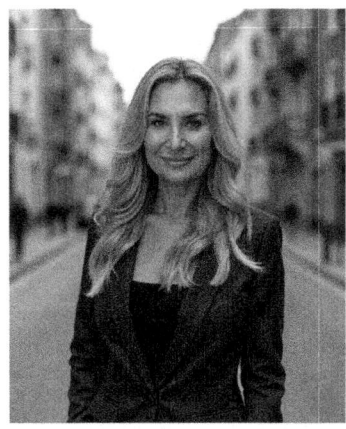

Kylie believes everyone holds the keys to unlocking their limitless potential. With a rich background in finance, business, nursing, herbal medicine, and mindset coaching, she has dedicated her life to empowering others. A certified HeartMath practitioner, Kylie combines the science of heart coherence with mindset strategies to inspire meaningful transformation. Drawing on her journey of overcoming challenges, Kylie connects with readers through her resilience and innovative thinking.

RECOMMENDATIONS

A Course in Miracles, Helen Schucman

Ancient Lotus Chant, Nikko Hansen

Biology of Belief, Bruce H Lipton

Breaking the Habit of Being Yourself, Dr Joe Dispenza

Gene Keys, Richard Rudd

The Divine Matrix, Gregg Braden

Heart Math Institute https://www.heartmath.org/

https://med.virginia.edu/perceptual-studies/our-research/

Journey of Souls, Dr Michael Newton

Letting Go: The Pathway of Surrender, Dr David Hawkins

The 5 Love Languages, Gary Chapman

The Field: The Quest for the Secret Force of the Universe, Lynne McTaggart

German New Medicine https://www.learninggnm.com/

The Hidden Messages in Water, Dr. Masaru Emoto

Reality Transurfing Steps 1–5, Vadim Zeland

Return to Life: Extraordinary Cases of Children Who Remember Past Lives, Dr Jim Tucker

Source the film, https://sourcethefilm.org/

The Lotus Sutra: https://www.youtube.com/watch?v=r364h19dXio

University of Virginia studies on reincarnation and consciousness

REFERENCES

Albini, F. & Riva, M. A. (2020) *Medicus curat: Sungazing versus spectacles?* Eye (London). [Online] 34 (8), 1303–1304.

Austin, V. (2020) *The secret intelligence of water: Macroscopic evidence of water responding to human consciousness.* United States: Lifestyle Entrepreneurs Press.

CIA (1983) *Analysis and assessment of gateway process.* Available at: https://www.cia.gov/readingroom/document/cia-rdp96-00788r001700210040-8 (Accessed: 17 January 2025).

Consciousness Calibrations (2022). *Map of spiritual progress.* Available at: https://consciousnesscalibrations.com/map-of-spiritual-progress/ (Accessed: 27 December 2024).

Eriksson, P.S., Perfilieva, E., Björk-Eriksson, T., Alborn, A.M., Nordborg, C., Peterson, D.A. and Gage, F.H. (1998) Neurogenesis in the adult human hippocampus, *Nature Medicine*, 4(11), pp. 1313–1317.

Johns Hopkins Medicine (2024). *Forgiveness: Your health depends on it.* Available at: https://www.hopkinsmedicine.org/health/wellness-and-prevention/forgiveness-your-health-depends-on-it Accessed 12 December 2024).

Lorber, J. (1980) Is your brain really necessary?, *Scientific American*, 242(6), 22–29. Available at: https://www.scientificamerican.com (Accessed: 9 January 2025).

Matos, M., Santos, I.M., Gonçalves, M.A., & Pereira, A. (2021). Biofield therapies and their connection to energy medicine: A review. *International Journal of Healing and Caring, 21*(3), 15-25.

Mead, M.N. (2008) Benefits of sunlight: A bright spot for human health, Environmental health perspectives. Available at: https://pmc.ncbi.nlm.nih.gov/articles/PMC2290997/ (Accessed: 12 December 2024).

Pfaff, D. W., Ribeiro, A. C., Matthews, J. R., & Kow, L. M. (2008). *Arousal: How your brain is wired for behavior.* Harvard University Press.

Three Initiates, 1908. *The Kybalion: A study of the Hermetic philosophy of Ancient Egypt and Greece.* Chicago: Yogi Publication Society.

Wade, K.A., Garry, M., Read, J.D. and Lindsay, D.S. (2002). A picture is worth a thousand lies: Using false photographs to create false childhood memories, *Psychonomic Bulletin & Review*, 9(3), pp. 597–603. Available at: https://www.bbc.com/news/science-environment-24286258 (Accessed: 9 December 2024).

Worthington, E. L. & Scherer, M. (2004) Forgiveness is an emotion-focused coping strategy that can reduce health risks and promote health resilience: theory, review, and hypotheses. *Psychology & Health.* [Online] 19(3), 385–405.

Zimmermann, M. (1986) 'Neurophysiology of Sensory Systems', in *Fundamentals of Sensory Physiology.* Berlin: Springer, pp. 68–69.

Printed in Great Britain
by Amazon